M000305178

100 Fitness Challenges

2020

Neila Rey | darebee.com

Copyright ©Darebee, 2020. All rights reserved.

No part of this publication may be reproduced, distributed, or transmitted
in any form or by any means, including photocopying, recording, or other electronic or mechanical methods,
without the prior written permission of the publisher, except in the case of brief quotations embodied in
critical reviews and certain other noncommercial uses permitted by copyright law.

First Printing, 2020.
ISBN 13: 978-1-84481-155-7
ISBN 10: 1-84481-155-7

Warning and Disclaimer
Although every precaution has been taken to verify the accuracy of the information contained herein, the
author and publisher assume no responsibility for any errors or omissions. No liability is assumed for damage
or injury that may result from the use of information contained within.

# Thank you!

Thank you for purchasing 100 Challenges, DAREBEE project print edition. DAREBEE is a non-profit global fitness resource dedicated to making fitness accessible for everyone, no matter their circumstances. The project is supported exclusively via user donations and paperback royalties.

After printing costs and store fees every book developed by the DAREBEE project makes $1 and it goes directly into our project maintenance and development fund.

Each sale helps us keep the DAREBEE resource growing, maintain it and keep it up. Thank you for making a difference in its future!

**Other books in this series include:**

100 No-Equipment Workouts Vol 1.
100 No-Equipment Workouts Vol 2.
100 No-Equipment Workouts Vol 3.
100 Office Workouts
Pocket Workouts: 100 no-equipment workouts
ABS 100 Workouts: Visual Easy-To-Follow ABS Exercise Routines for All Fitness Levels

Fitness is a journey, not a destination.
**Darebee Project**

## About The Author

Neila Rey is the founder of Darebee, a global fitness resource. She is committed to democratizing fitness by removing the barriers to it and increasing accessibility. Every workout published in her books utilizes the latest in exercise science and has undergone thorough field testing and refinement through Darebee volunteers. When she's not busy running Darebee she is focused on finding fresh ways to make exercise easier and more enjoyable.

# 100 challenges

1. 1 Minute Meditation
2. 1 Minute Plank
3. 1 Minute Yoga
4. 2 Minute Abs
5. 10k Crunches
6. 10k Half Jacks
7. 10k Jacks
8. 10k Punches
9. 10k Squats
10. 15 Days Of Fitness
11. 30 Days Of Fitness
12. 20k High Knees
13. 50 Burpees A Day
14. 50 Push-Ups A Day
15. 50 Squats A Day
16. 100 Burpees A Day
17. 100
18. 1000 Push-Ups
19. Ab
20. Ab  Level 2
21. Ab Advanced
22. Abs And Core
23. Abs Of Steel
24. Action Hero
25. Back & Shoulders
26. Balance
27. Boxer
28. Burpee
29. Calves Of Steel
30. Cardio & Abs
31. Cardio Blast
32. Cardio
33. Cardio HIIT
34. Chest And Arms
35. Core
36. Core Control
37. Daily Gratitude
38. Dead Hang
39. De-Stress
40. Endurance
41. Everest
42. Fiber
43. First Thing Water
44. Five Minute Plank
45. Flex
46. Flex Hang
47. Get To Bed On Time
48. Gladiator
49. Good Morning
50. Hollow Hold
51. Home Marathon
52. Homerun
53. Impact
54. Impossible Abs
55. Iron Core
56. Iron Glutes
57. Iron Will
58. Jump Rope
59. Kicks & Punches
60. Knee Push-Ups
61. Legs Of Steel
62. Makeover
63. Meditation
64. Micro HIIT
65. Multiplank
66. Negative Pull-Up
67. Ninja
68. No Junk Food
69. No Salt
70. No Sugar
71. Office
72. Only Homemade
73. Plank
74. Plant Based
75. Posture
76. Power Grip
77. Power Pull
78. Power Walk
79. Pull-Up
80. Pull-Up Level 2
81. Punches & Squats
82. Punch Out
83. Push-Up Ladder
84. Push-Up Master
85. Salad A Day
86. Spartan
87. Splits
88. Squats & Punches
89. Squats
90. Squats Push-Ups
91. Target 10
92. Touch Your Toes
93. Tricep Dips
94. Upper Body
95. Upper Body Light
96. Upper Body Plus
97. Walkabout
98. Wall Push-Ups
99. Wall-Sit
100. Yoga Abs

# Introduction

Fitness is a puzzle of two halves. One part is unavoidably physical. The other part, however is mental. We now know that the central nervous system spreads across the entire body and distributes some of its processing power in places like the stomach and the heart. This makes the mind an integral part of getting fit and getting fit now affects our mental as well as our physical health.

This 100 Fitness Challenges workbook then is more than just a collection of physical activities that will exercise your body. By giving you specific, month-long daily tasks to perform it creates for you an easy-to-follow routine that has equal physical, mental and psychological components that will transform you inside and out.

The science on micro-workouts has been in for some time. It shows that persistent, consistent physical work creates adaptive responses in the body that deliver the kind of physical transformation that makes us fitter and healthier. Persistent, consistent physical work like the exercise you have to perform in this 100 Fitness Challenges workbook also create deeper changes at a mental level.

The ability to stick to a daily routine for a month changes how our brain handles pressure and helps enhance our sense of discipline and our ability to focus. Discipline and focus, in turn, change our motivation. Motivation is what helps us do things, consistently, that benefit us.

So, one 100 Fitness Challenges, collectively, represent over eight years' worth of sustained physical activity. Were you to do them all, one after the other, you would end up a totally different person at the end of it, both in the way you control your body and the way you run your mind.

Go, ahead. Dive in. Pick one and start and begin your journey to your better self.

# The Manual

This book contains approximately 3,000 days worth of physical and mental challenges that will transform your body and mind. How you start is up to you. You could start from challenge one and try to do them all consecutively. Or, you could just dip in and pick one at random each month until you have exhausted every challenge in this workbook.

You can cross out each day on the page, as you do it. This becomes a visual record of your fitness journey and helps motivate you further.

Most of the exercises you have to do are intuitive and easy to understand. There are, however, instructions at the beginning of each challenge that will better help you understand what it is you need to do. Some of the benefits you will gain are also mentioned there.

If you are in doubt about some exercise you can check out our online video exercise library at: **http://darebee.com/exercises.**

Fitness is a gift you give your future self.
Darebee Project

# 1  1 Minute Meditation

Rewire your brain and improve your life: take a moment to meditate! It'll only take a minute.

Find a comfortable and quite place, close your eyes and begin. Use the timer below to control your breathing. Adjust the volume on your device and press "start" to begin a guided session.

Instructions: Inhale through the nose for 4 seconds, hold your breath for 7 seconds and then exhale for 8 seconds.

# 1 minute meditation

## 30-DAY CHALLENGE

© darebee.com

| 1 Done! | 2 Done! | 3 Done! | 4 Done! | 5 Done! |
|---|---|---|---|---|
| 6 Done! | 7 Done! | 8 Done! | 9 Done! | 10 Done! |
| 11 Done! | 12 Done! | 13 Done! | 14 Done! | 15 Done! |
| 16 Done! | 17 Done! | 18 Done! | 19 Done! | 20 Done! |
| 21 Done! | 22 Done! | 23 Done! | 24 Done! | 25 Done! |
| 26 Done! | 27 Done! | 28 Done! | 29 Done! | 30 Done! |

## 2     1 Minute Plank

We all know we need a strong core. This is why we should start each day chopping down trees, swinging from trapezes, walking along monorails, balancing on high wires and doing backflips on balance beams. Or ... we could perhaps devote a minute a day. Every day, for a month. And get the strong core we deserve.

Instructions: Hold a plank for 60 seconds every day for 30 days. Split the total minute into manageable sets if you have to.

# 1-minute plank

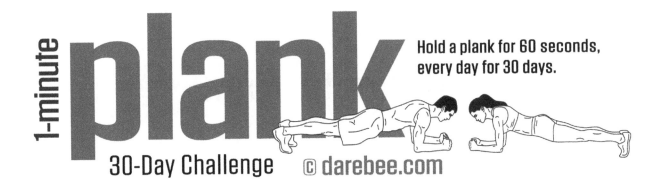

**Hold a plank for 60 seconds, every day for 30 days.**

30-Day Challenge  © darebee.com

| | | | | |
|---|---|---|---|---|
| **1** Done! | **2** Done! | **3** Done! | **4** Done! | **5** Done! |
| **6** Done! | **7** Done! | **8** Done! | **9** Done! | **10** Done! |
| **11** Done! | **12** Done! | **13** Done! | **14** Done! | **15** Done! |
| **16** Done! | **17** Done! | **18** Done! | **19** Done! | **20** Done! |
| **21** Done! | **22** Done! | **23** Done! | **24** Done! | **25** Done! |
| **26** Done! | **27** Done! | **28** Done! | **29** Done! | **30** Done! |

# 3    1 Minute Yoga

If you only have 60 seconds a day to devote to training then the one-minute, 30-day Yoga Challenge will help you make the most of it. The secret to getting results in your physical training is consistency and perseverance and over 30 days you will learn that even a small amount of time, spent correctly can make a huge difference.

# 1 min YOGA

## 30-Day Challenge

Hold the pose of the day for 60 seconds in total.

© darebee.com

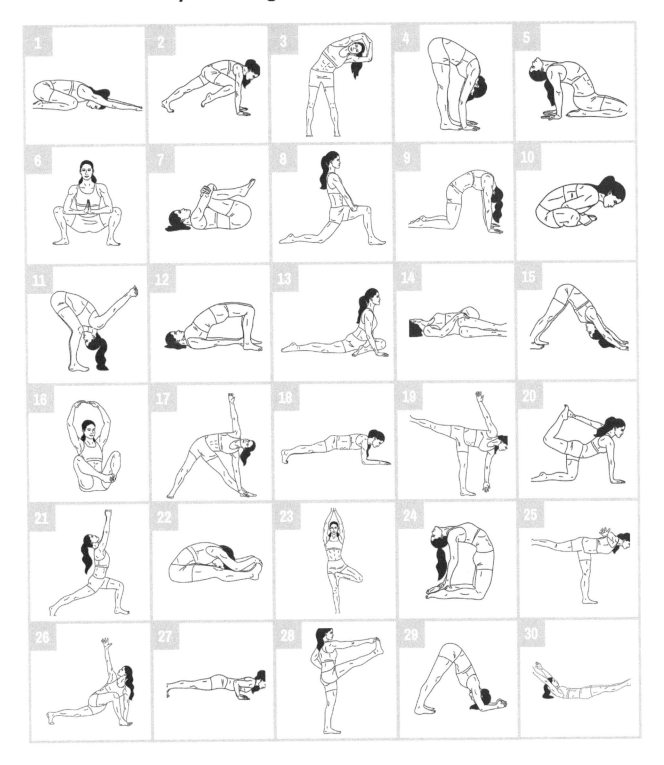

# 4    2 Minute Abs

Strong abs help you sit, stand, walk, run and jump better. They take the load off your spine and can help reduce the incidence of back pain associated with modern living and long periods of sitting down at work.

Split 2 minutes into manageable sets when, and if, you need to. The time is given in total so, for example, holding a side plank for 2 minutes = 1 minute per side.

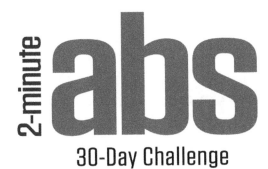

# 2-minute abs
## 30-Day Challenge

Repeat the exercises
for each day for 2 minutes,
every day for 30 days.

© darebee.com

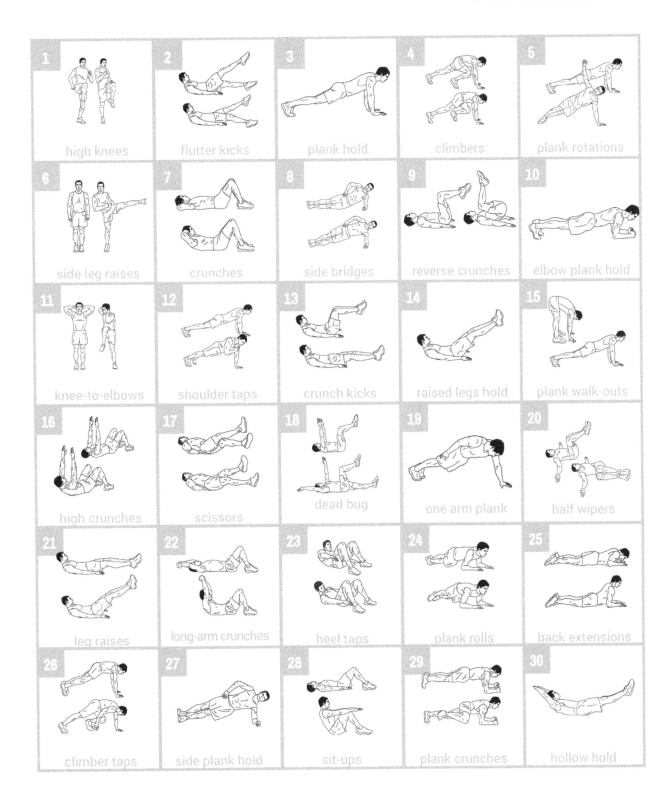

| | | | | |
|---|---|---|---|---|
| **1** high knees | **2** flutter kicks | **3** plank hold | **4** climbers | **5** plank rotations |
| **6** side leg raises | **7** crunches | **8** side bridges | **9** reverse crunches | **10** elbow plank hold |
| **11** knee-to-elbows | **12** shoulder taps | **13** crunch kicks | **14** raised legs hold | **15** plank walk-outs |
| **16** high crunches | **17** scissors | **18** dead bug | **19** one arm plank | **20** half wipers |
| **21** leg raises | **22** long-arm crunches | **23** heel taps | **24** plank rolls | **25** back extensions |
| **26** climber taps | **27** side plank hold | **28** sit-ups | **29** plank crunches | **30** hollow hold |

## 5   10k Crunches

Muscles trigger their adaptive response and become stronger and more capable in direct response to perceived need. The 10,000 Crunches Challenge creates the perceived need necessary, one day at a time.

You can choose to do all the crunches in one go or separate them into chunks and either do them in installments in one single training session or do them in chunks, throughout the day. The goal is to get to the total number required by the end of the day.

# 10,000

**CRUNCHES**

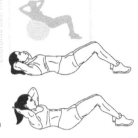

split total reps into manageable sets © darebee.com

| | | | | |
|---|---|---|---|---|
| **1** 140 crunches | **2** 160 crunches | **3** 200 crunches | **4** 100 crunches | **5** 200 crunches |
| **6** 220 crunches | **7** 260 crunches | **8** 100 crunches | **9** 300 crunches | **10** 320 crunches |
| **11** 360 crunches | **12** 100 crunches | **13** 400 crunches | **14** 420 crunches | **15** 460 crunches |
| **16** 100 crunches | **17** 460 crunches | **18** 480 crunches | **19** 500 crunches | **20** 100 crunches |
| **21** 500 crunches | **22** 520 crunches | **23** 540 crunches | **24** 100 crunches | **25** 540 crunches |
| **26** 560 crunches | **27** 580 crunches | **28** 100 crunches | **29** 580 crunches | **30** 600 crunches |

## 6    10k Half Jacks

Half Jacks are a quick, easy exercise that activates your cardiovascular system, gets your lungs working and challenges your fascial fitness. Because they work both lower and upper body Half Jacks contribute to overall coordination and balance and even help develop a stronger core.

You can do the Half Jacks, each day, all in one go or you can choose to do them in brief installments in one session or chunk them up and do them in lots throughout the day. Your goal is to finish the day having completed the overall number of Half Jacks required.

# 10,000

30-DAY CHALLENGE **HALF-JACKS** split total reps into manageable sets © darebee.com

| | | | | |
|---|---|---|---|---|
| **1** 70 half-jacks | **2** 80 half-jacks | **3** 100 half-jacks | **4** 150 half-jacks | **5** 100 half-jacks |
| **6** 200 half-jacks | **7** 250 half-jacks | **8** 300 half-jacks | **9** 400 half-jacks | **10** 100 half-jacks |
| **11** 400 half-jacks | **12** 450 half-jacks | **13** 500 half-jacks | **14** 550 half-jacks | **15** 100 half-jacks |
| **16** 400 half-jacks | **17** 450 half-jacks | **18** 500 half-jacks | **19** 550 half-jacks | **20** 100 half-jacks |
| **21** 300 half-jacks | **22** 500 half-jacks | **23** 200 half-jacks | **24** 300 half-jacks | **25** 100 half-jacks |
| **26** 400 half-jacks | **27** 500 half-jacks | **28** 600 half-jacks | **29** 650 half-jacks | **30** 700 half-jacks |

# 7    10k Jacks

Jacks are a moderate-impact exercise that will raise your body's core temperature, get your lungs working, help develop better fascial fitness and improve your cardiovascular capability. The 10,000 Jacks challenge will help you elevate your overall fitness and contribute to your ability to better control your body.

You can choose to do all the Jacks required, each day, in one go. You can do them in installments in one workout where you take breaks in-between. Or, you can do them in chunks of physical activity throughout the day. The goal is to complete, each day, the total number of Jacks required.

# 10,000

**30-DAY CHALLENGE**   **JUMPING JACKS**

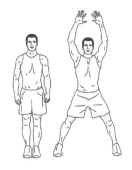

split total reps
into manageable sets

© darebee.com

| | | | | |
|---|---|---|---|---|
| **1** 160 jumping jacks | **2** 180 jumping jacks | **3** 200 jumping jacks | **4** 100 jumping jacks | **5** 220 jumping jacks |
| **6** 240 jumping jacks | **7** 280 jumping jacks | **8** 100 jumping jacks | **9** 300 jumping jacks | **10** 320 jumping jacks |
| **11** 340 jumping jacks | **12** 100 jumping jacks | **13** 360 jumping jacks | **14** 380 jumping jacks | **15** 400 jumping jacks |
| **16** 100 jumping jacks | **17** 420 jumping jacks | **18** 440 jumping jacks | **19** 460 jumping jacks | **20** 100 jumping jacks |
| **21** 480 jumping jacks | **22** 500 jumping jacks | **23** 540 jumping jacks | **24** 100 jumping jacks | **25** 560 jumping jacks |
| **26** 580 jumping jacks | **27** 600 jumping jacks | **28** 100 jumping jacks | **29** 640 jumping jacks | **30** 700 jumping jacks |

# 8    10k Punches

Each day consists of a total number of reps. You split the total into manageable sets but there is a twist - before every set you have to do 5 push-ups. It doesn't matter how many sets you split the total into if you break and rest, it counts as a full set and before your next go you have to do 5 push-ups. Every 4th day is an easy day with only 100 punches in total for the day. Each punch counts as one rep.

# 10,000

## 30-DAY CHALLENGE

**PUNCHES** 5 push-ups before every set © darebee.com

| | | | | |
|---|---|---|---|---|
| **1**<br>160<br>punches | **2**<br>180<br>punches | **3**<br>200<br>punches | **4**<br>100<br>punches | **5**<br>220<br>punches |
| **6**<br>240<br>punches | **7**<br>280<br>punches | **8**<br>100<br>punches | **9**<br>300<br>punches | **10**<br>320<br>punches |
| **11**<br>340<br>punches | **12**<br>100<br>punches | **13**<br>360<br>punches | **14**<br>380<br>punches | **15**<br>400<br>punches |
| **16**<br>100<br>punches | **17**<br>420<br>punches | **18**<br>440<br>punches | **19**<br>460<br>punches | **20**<br>100<br>punches |
| **21**<br>480<br>punches | **22**<br>500<br>punches | **23**<br>540<br>punches | **24**<br>100<br>punches | **25**<br>560<br>punches |
| **26**<br>580<br>punches | **27**<br>600<br>punches | **28**<br>100<br>punches | **29**<br>640<br>punches | **30**<br>700<br>punches |

## 9  10k Squats

Squats target the quads which are the single largest muscle group in the body. They, in turn, make a sizeable oxygen demand on the body which helps develop better aerobic fitness. In addition, they help develop core stability and the stability of the knee joint.

You can do all of the required number of squats, each day, in one go. You can choose to do them in short installments in one training session, taking some breaks in between. Or, you can do them in installments throughout the day. The goal, always, is to finish the day with the required number of squats completed.

# 10,000

30-DAY CHALLENGE **SQUATS** split total reps into manageable sets © darebee.com

| | | | | |
|---|---|---|---|---|
| **1** 100 squats | **2** 140 squats | **3** 160 squats | **4** 200 squats | **5** 220 squats |
| **6** 240 squats | **7** 260 squats | **8** 200 squats | **9** 280 squats | **10** 300 squats |
| **11** 320 squats | **12** 200 squats | **13** 340 squats | **14** 360 squats | **15** 380 squats |
| **16** 200 squats | **17** 400 squats | **18** 420 squats | **19** 440 squats | **20** 200 squats |
| **21** 460 squats | **22** 480 squats | **23** 500 squats | **24** 200 squats | **25** 520 squats |
| **26** 540 squats | **27** 560 squats | **28** 200 squats | **29** 580 squats | **30** 600 squats |

# 10    15 Days Of Fitness

Fitness means being able to move your body as you will. Exercising each day, no matter what shape or form that takes, is a key requirement to forming the habit that will help you achieve your fitness goals.

This is a short commitment, lasting over fifteen days, that asks you to do something physical each day. In return you begin to get into the habit and discipline of doing something physical each day.

# 15 Days of Fitness

## CHALLENGE

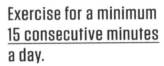

Exercise for a minimum 15 consecutive minutes a day.

© darebee.com

| 1 | 2 | 3 | 4 | 5 |
|---|---|---|---|---|
| I exercised today! | I exercised today! | I exercised today! | I exercised today! | I exercised today! |
| **6** | **7** | **8** | **9** | **10** |
| I exercised today! | I exercised today! | I exercised today! | I exercised today! | I exercised today! |
| **11** | **12** | **13** | **14** | **15** |
| I exercised today! | I exercised today! | I exercised today! | I exercised today! | I exercised today! |

## 11    30 Days Of Fitness

Doing something physical over 30 days is going to help you change not just your body but also your mind. Motivation requires a clear understanding of goals and purpose. Clearly defined goals and purpose deliver the consistent approach to exercise that is perceived as discipline.

The 30 Days of Fitness challenge will transform you inside and out. Plus, it is a key component to learning how to build and maintain momentum in your fitness journey.

# 30 Days of Fitness

## CHALLENGE

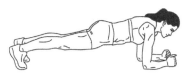

Exercise for a minimum **15 consecutive minutes** a day

© darebee.com

| 1 | 2 | 3 | 4 | 5 |
|---|---|---|---|---|
| I exercised today! | I exercised today! | I exercised today! | I exercised today! | I exercised today! |
| **6** | **7** | **8** | **9** | **10** |
| I exercised today! | I exercised today! | I exercised today! | I exercised today! | I exercised today! |
| **11** | **12** | **13** | **14** | **15** |
| I exercised today! | I exercised today! | I exercised today! | I exercised today! | I exercised today! |
| **16** | **17** | **18** | **19** | **20** |
| I exercised today! | I exercised today! | I exercised today! | I exercised today! | I exercised today! |
| **21** | **22** | **23** | **24** | **25** |
| I exercised today! | I exercised today! | I exercised today! | I exercised today! | I exercised today! |
| **26** | **27** | **28** | **29** | **30** |
| I exercised today! | I exercised today! | I exercised today! | I exercised today! | I exercised today! |

## 12    20k High Knees

High Knees are a moderate impact exercise that also targets calves, tendons and glutes alongside the quads. The high-oxygen consumption generated by it also forces your heart and lungs work harder, helping you develop better aerobic and cardiovascular fitness.

Aim to bring your knee, each time, to the height of your waist. Do all of the required High Knees each day in one go or, break them down into installments you can do in one training session with breaks or throughout the day.

# 20,000

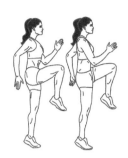

**30-DAY CHALLENGE** **HIGH KNEES** split total reps into manageable sets © **darebee.com**

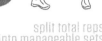
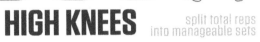

| | | | | |
|---|---|---|---|---|
| **1**<br>**200**<br>high knees | **2**<br>**400**<br>high knees | **3**<br>**200**<br>high knees | **4**<br>**500**<br>high knees | **5**<br>**200**<br>high knees |
| **6**<br>**600**<br>high knees | **7**<br>**200**<br>high knees | **8**<br>**700**<br>high knees | **9**<br>**200**<br>high knees | **10**<br>**800**<br>high knees |
| **11**<br>**200**<br>high knees | **12**<br>**900**<br>high knees | **13**<br>**200**<br>high knees | **14**<br>**1000**<br>high knees | **15**<br>**200**<br>high knees |
| **16**<br>**1100**<br>high knees | **17**<br>**200**<br>high knees | **18**<br>**1200**<br>high knees | **19**<br>**200**<br>high knees | **20**<br>**1300**<br>high knees |
| **21**<br>**200**<br>high knees | **22**<br>**1400**<br>high knees | **23**<br>**200**<br>high knees | **24**<br>**1600**<br>high knees | **25**<br>**200**<br>high knees |
| **26**<br>**1700**<br>high knees | **27**<br>**200**<br>high knees | **28**<br>**1800**<br>high knees | **29**<br>**200**<br>high knees | **30**<br>**2000**<br>high knees |

## 13    50 Burpees A Day

Your body is your ball and chain. Its mass drags you down, keeps you pinned to the planet. Everything you do is a fight against the planet's gravity well. Just like a ball and chain, smartly used, can become an awesome weapon so can your body be transformed into an instrument of your will. All you need to do is beat the planet's gravity by training your muscles to work with more than just the load of your body. You guessed where this is leading. Burpees are your best bet here. They become your bud for a month as you teach your muscles to make light work of your body's mass.

EXTRA CREDIT: do in one workout, up to 20 second breaks are ok.
EXTRA EXTRA CREDIT: do a full burpee with a push-up.

# 50 BURPEES
## IN ONE GO

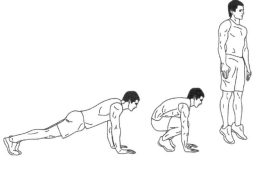

CHALLENGE

© darebee.com

| | | | | |
|---|---|---|---|---|
| **1** Done! | **2** Done! | **3** Done! | **4** Done! | **5** Done! |
| **6** Done! | **7** Done! | **8** Done! | **9** Done! | **10** Done! |
| **11** Done! | **12** Done! | **13** Done! | **14** Done! | **15** Done! |
| **16** Done! | **17** Done! | **18** Done! | **19** Done! | **20** Done! |
| **21** Done! | **22** Done! | **23** Done! | **24** Done! | **25** Done! |
| **26** Done! | **27** Done! | **28** Done! | **29** Done! | **30** Done! |

## 14   50 Push-Ups A Day

Transform your body, change your mind, develop discipline, feel differently about yourself and the world. And that is not even the sum total of the benefits to be reaped by doing the 50 Push-Ups a Day Challenge. Do them all at once. Do them in sets of 5 or 10 at a time. Do them all within an hour or space them out throughout the day. It doesn't matter how you decide to do them as long as you actually do 50 push-ups a day, every day for a month. The transformation is something you will feel yourself.

EXTRA CREDIT: Complete every day before breakfast.

# 50 Push-Ups a Day

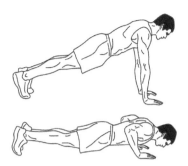

**CHALLENGE** Split into manageable sets.
Extra Credit: complete before breakfast

© darebee.com

| | | | | |
|---|---|---|---|---|
| **1** Done! | **2** Done! | **3** Done! | **4** Done! | **5** Done! |
| **6** Done! | **7** Done! | **8** Done! | **9** Done! | **10** Done! |
| **11** Done! | **12** Done! | **13** Done! | **14** Done! | **15** Done! |
| **16** Done! | **17** Done! | **18** Done! | **19** Done! | **20** Done! |
| **21** Done! | **22** Done! | **23** Done! | **24** Done! | **25** Done! |
| **26** Done! | **27** Done! | **28** Done! | **29** Done! | **30** Done! |

# 15    50 Squats A Day

Repetitive, low intensity, daily exercise helps build a sound foundation for your fitness. Fifty squats each day may not sound like a lot but if you do that every day, for a month you introduce a constant load that triggers the adaptive response that will change you physically.

Add to it the fact that the mental focus required to do this every day also changes you mentally and you have an easy inside & out, workout program.

EXTRA CREDIT: Complete every day before breakfast.

# 50 SQUATS A DAY

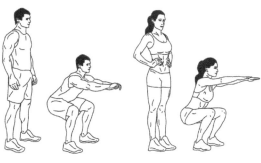

**CHALLENGE** Split into manageable sets.
Extra Credit: complete before breakfast

© darebee.com

| | | | | |
|---|---|---|---|---|
| **1** Done! | **2** Done! | **3** Done! | **4** Done! | **5** Done! |
| **6** Done! | **7** Done! | **8** Done! | **9** Done! | **10** Done! |
| **11** Done! | **12** Done! | **13** Done! | **14** Done! | **15** Done! |
| **16** Done! | **17** Done! | **18** Done! | **19** Done! | **20** Done! |
| **21** Done! | **22** Done! | **23** Done! | **24** Done! | **25** Done! |
| **26** Done! | **27** Done! | **28** Done! | **29** Done! | **30** Done! |

## 16    100 Burpees A Day

Your body is your ball and chain. Its mass drags you down, keeps you pinned to the planet. Everything you do is a fight against the planet's gravity well. Just like a ball and chain, smartly used, can become an awesome weapon so can your body be transformed into an instrument of your will. All you need to do is beat the planet's gravity by training your muscles to work with more than just the load of your body. You guessed where this is leading. Burpees are your best bet here. They become your bud for a month as you teach your muscles to make light work of your body's mass.

EXTRA CREDIT: do in one workout, up to 30 second breaks are ok.
EXTRA EXTRA CREDIT: do a full burpee with a push-up.

# 100 Burpees a Day

**CHALLENGE** Split into manageable sets.

© darebee.com

| | | | | |
|---|---|---|---|---|
| **1** Done! | **2** Done! | **3** Done! | **4** Done! | **5** Done! |
| **6** Done! | **7** Done! | **8** Done! | **9** Done! | **10** Done! |
| **11** Done! | **12** Done! | **13** Done! | **14** Done! | **15** Done! |
| **16** Done! | **17** Done! | **18** Done! | **19** Done! | **20** Done! |
| **21** Done! | **22** Done! | **23** Done! | **24** Done! | **25** Done! |
| **26** Done! | **27** Done! | **28** Done! | **29** Done! | **30** Done! |

## 17 100

One hundred reps of something different every day is a shocker to the body and mind. It will move you out of your comfort zone, challenge your muscles to respond by getting stronger and your mind to stay focused so you can get through this month.

You can perform all 100 reps in one go or you can take short breaks as you do them or you can chunk them into installments and perform them throughout the day. The goal, however, is to complete all 100 reps of each exercise shown in one day.

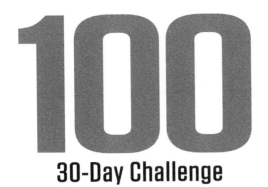

# 100

## 30-Day Challenge

**Repeat each exercise 100 times.**
Split into manageable sets
**Extra Credit:** in one go

ⓒ **darebee.com**

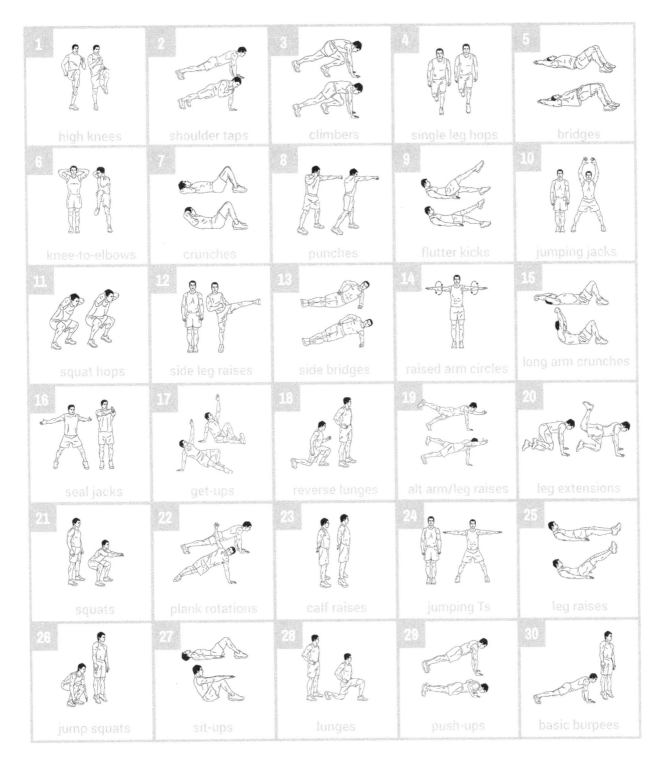

| | | | | |
|---|---|---|---|---|
| 1 high knees | 2 shoulder taps | 3 climbers | 4 single leg hops | 5 bridges |
| 6 knee-to-elbows | 7 crunches | 8 punches | 9 flutter kicks | 10 jumping jacks |
| 11 squat hops | 12 side leg raises | 13 side bridges | 14 raised arm circles | 15 long arm crunches |
| 16 seal jacks | 17 get-ups | 18 reverse lunges | 19 alt arm/leg raises | 20 leg extensions |
| 21 squats | 22 plank rotations | 23 calf raises | 24 jumping Ts | 25 leg raises |
| 26 jump squats | 27 sit-ups | 28 lunges | 29 push-ups | 30 basic burpees |

# 18    1000 Push-Ups

Push-ups are a closed kinetic chain exercise which means they generate a large reaction force at the wrist, elbow and shoulder joints. This helps your upper body strength and overall bone density which promotes both mental and physical health.

You can do each day's required rep number all in one go. You can break it up into chunks and take breaks in-between. Or, you can spread the load throughout the day. The goal is to finish the day with the required number of push-ups completed.

# 1,000

## 30-DAY CHALLENGE  PUSH-UPS

split total reps
into manageable sets  © darebee.com

| 1 | 2 | 3 | 4 | 5 |
|---|---|---|---|---|
| **30** push-ups | 10sec plank 2 times a day | **35** push-ups | 10sec plank 3 times a day | **40** push-ups |

| 6 | 7 | 8 | 9 | 10 |
|---|---|---|---|---|
| 20sec plank 2 times a day | **45** push-ups | 20sec plank 3 times a day | **50** push-ups | 25sec plank 2 times a day |

| 11 | 12 | 13 | 14 | 15 |
|---|---|---|---|---|
| **55** push-ups | 25sec plank 3 times a day | **60** push-ups | 30sec plank 2 times a day | **65** push-ups |

| 16 | 17 | 18 | 19 | 20 |
|---|---|---|---|---|
| 30sec plank 3 times a day | **70** push-ups | 35sec plank 2 times a day | **75** push-ups | 35sec plank 3 times a day |

| 21 | 22 | 23 | 24 | 25 |
|---|---|---|---|---|
| **80** push-ups | 40sec plank 2 times a day | **85** push-ups | 40sec plank 3 times a day | **90** push-ups |

| 26 | 27 | 28 | 29 | 30 |
|---|---|---|---|---|
| 45sec plank 2 times a day | **100** push-ups | 60sec plank 2 times a day | **120** push-ups | 60sec plank 3 times a day |

## 19 Abs

Strong abs support the body, reduce overall muscle fatigue during exercise and help you sit, stand, walk, run, jump and kick better. Building strong abs requires persistence and dedication.

Each day of the Abs Challenge consists of three distinct exercises that will challenge each of the four abdominal muscle groups. You can do them separately at different times in the day or you can do them all in one go or you can take small breaks in between to help you recover. The goal is to finish the day having met the requirements set out.

# ab

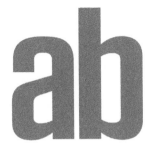
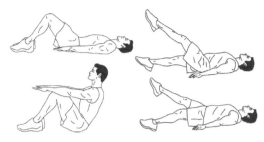

**30-DAY CHALLENGE**

split total reps
into manageable sets

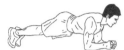

© darebee.com

| | | | | |
|---|---|---|---|---|
| **1**<br>10 sit-ups<br>20 flutter kicks<br>30sec plank | **2**<br>14 sit-ups<br>40 flutter kicks<br>40sec plank | **3**<br>16 sit-ups<br>60 flutter kicks<br>45sec plank | **4**<br>20 sit-ups<br>20 flutter kicks<br>20sec plank | **5**<br>24 sit-ups<br>80 flutter kicks<br>50sec plank |
| **6**<br>26 sit-ups<br>100 flutter kicks<br>1min plank | **7**<br>28 sit-ups<br>110 flutter kicks<br>1min10sec plank | **8**<br>20 sit-ups<br>20 flutter kicks<br>20sec plank | **9**<br>30 sit-ups<br>120 flutter kicks<br>1min20sec plank | **10**<br>32 sit-ups<br>130 flutter kicks<br>1min30sec plank |
| **11**<br>34 sit-ups<br>140 flutter kicks<br>1min40sec plank | **12**<br>20 sit-ups<br>20 flutter kicks<br>20sec plank | **13**<br>36 sit-ups<br>150 flutter kicks<br>1min45sec plank | **14**<br>38 sit-ups<br>160 flutter kicks<br>1min50sec plank | **15**<br>40 sit-ups<br>180 flutter kicks<br>2min plank |
| **16**<br>20 sit-ups<br>20 flutter kicks<br>20sec plank | **17**<br>42 sit-ups<br>190 flutter kicks<br>2min10sec plank | **18**<br>44 sit-ups<br>200 flutter kicks<br>2min20sec plank | **19**<br>46 sit-ups<br>210 flutter kicks<br>2min30sec plank | **20**<br>20 sit-ups<br>20 flutter kicks<br>20sec plank |
| **21**<br>50 sit-ups<br>220 flutter kicks<br>2min40sec plank | **22**<br>52 sit-ups<br>230 flutter kicks<br>2min50sec plank | **23**<br>54 sit-ups<br>240 flutter kicks<br>3min plank | **24**<br>20 sit-ups<br>20 flutter kicks<br>20sec plank | **25**<br>60 sit-ups<br>250 flutter kicks<br>3min10sec plank |
| **26**<br>62 sit-ups<br>260 flutter kicks<br>3min20sec plank | **27**<br>64 sit-ups<br>280 flutter kicks<br>3min30sec plank | **28**<br>20 sit-ups<br>20 flutter kicks<br>20sec plank | **29**<br>68 sit-ups<br>290 flutter kicks<br>3min40sec plank | **30**<br>70 sit-ups<br>300 flutter kicks<br>4min plank |

# 20 Ab Level 2

If you completed the Abs Challenge then you know what's in store for you here. Each day has specific abs-specific training requirements. Yes. it is a little challenging but that's because this is a Challenge. Get through it and you're well on your way to levelling up.

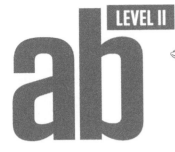
# ab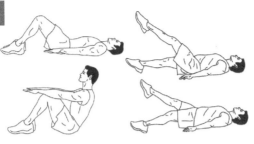

**LEVEL II**

**30-DAY CHALLENGE**

split total reps
into manageable sets

© darebee.com

| 1 | 2 | 3 | 4 | 5 |
|---|---|---|---|---|
| 40 sit-ups<br>60 flutter kicks<br>1min plank | 50 sit-ups<br>80 flutter kicks<br>1min20sec plank | 60 sit-ups<br>100 flutter kicks<br>1min plank x2sets | 40 sit-ups<br>60 flutter kicks<br>1min plank | 65 sit-ups<br>120 flutter kicks<br>1min40sec plank |
| **6** | **7** | **8** | **9** | **10** |
| 70 sit-ups<br>140 flutter kicks<br>2min plank | 75 sit-ups<br>160 flutter kicks<br>1min plank x3sets | 40 sit-ups<br>60 flutter kicks<br>1min plank | 80 sit-ups<br>180 flutter kicks<br>2min10sec plank | 85 sit-ups<br>200 flutter kicks<br>2min20sec plank |
| **11** | **12** | **13** | **14** | **15** |
| 90 sit-ups<br>220 flutter kicks<br>2min plank x2sets | 40 sit-ups<br>60 flutter kicks<br>1min plank | 95 sit-ups<br>240 flutter kicks<br>2min30sec plank | 100 sit-ups<br>260 flutter kicks<br>2min40sec plank | 105 sit-ups<br>280 flutter kicks<br>2min plank x3sets |
| **16** | **17** | **18** | **19** | **20** |
| 40 sit-ups<br>60 flutter kicks<br>1min plank | 110 sit-ups<br>300 flutter kicks<br>3min plank | 115 sit-ups<br>320 flutter kicks<br>3min10sec plank | 120 sit-ups<br>340 flutter kicks<br>2min plank x3sets | 40 sit-ups<br>60 flutter kicks<br>1min plank |
| **21** | **22** | **23** | **24** | **25** |
| 125 sit-ups<br>360 flutter kicks<br>3min20sec plank | 130 sit-ups<br>380 flutter kicks<br>3min40sec plank | 135 sit-ups<br>400 flutter kicks<br>2min plank x3sets | 40 sit-ups<br>60 flutter kicks<br>1min plank | 140 sit-ups<br>420 flutter kicks<br>4min plank |
| **26** | **27** | **28** | **29** | **30** |
| 145 sit-ups<br>440 flutter kicks<br>4min20sec plank | 150 sit-ups<br>460 flutter kicks<br>2min plank x4sets | 40 sit-ups<br>60 flutter kicks<br>1min plank | 155 sit-ups<br>480 flutter kicks<br>4min40sec plank | 160 sit-ups<br>500 flutter kicks<br>5min plank |

## 21 Ab Advanced

Abs advanced tackles all four major abs groups: External obliques (the muscles on the sides of the upper stomach), internal obliques (the muscles on the lower, outer part of the stomach), rectus abdominis (also popularly known as 'the six pack') and transverse abdominis (which are known as 'the core'). The result is an increase in overall sports performance, a higher resistance to fatigue and the ability to generate more power by having a better optimized upper/lower body kinetic chain.

# ab [ADVANCED]

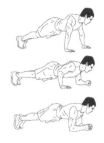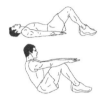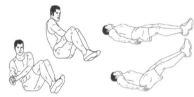

## 30-DAY CHALLENGE

split total reps
into manageable sets

© darebee.com

| | | | | |
|---|---|---|---|---|
| **1**<br>80 sit-ups<br>80 sitting twists<br>40 leg raises | **2**<br>120 sit-ups<br>120 sitting twists<br>60 leg raises | **3**<br>140 sit-ups<br>140 sitting twists<br>70 leg raises | **4**<br>**80**<br>up and down planks | **5**<br>160 sit-ups<br>160 sitting twists<br>80 leg raises |
| **6**<br>180 sit-ups<br>180 sitting twists<br>90 leg raises | **7**<br>200 sit-ups<br>200 sitting twists<br>100 leg raises | **8**<br>**100**<br>up and down planks | **9**<br>220 sit-ups<br>220 sitting twists<br>110 leg raises | **10**<br>240 sit-ups<br>240 sitting twists<br>120 leg raises |
| **11**<br>280 sit-ups<br>280 sitting twists<br>140 leg raises | **12**<br>**120**<br>up and down planks | **13**<br>300 sit-ups<br>300 sitting twists<br>150 leg raises | **14**<br>320 sit-ups<br>320 sitting twists<br>160 leg raises | **15**<br>340 sit-ups<br>340 sitting twists<br>170 leg raises |
| **16**<br>**140**<br>up and down planks | **17**<br>360 sit-ups<br>360 sitting twists<br>180 leg raises | **18**<br>380 sit-ups<br>380 sitting twists<br>190 leg raises | **19**<br>400 sit-ups<br>400 sitting twists<br>200 leg raises | **20**<br>**160**<br>up and down planks |
| **21**<br>420 sit-ups<br>420 sitting twists<br>210 leg raises | **22**<br>440 sit-ups<br>440 sitting twists<br>220 leg raises | **23**<br>460 sit-ups<br>460 sitting twists<br>230 leg raises | **24**<br>**180**<br>up and down planks | **25**<br>500 sit-ups<br>500 sitting twists<br>250 leg raises |
| **26**<br>520 sit-ups<br>520 sitting twists<br>260 leg raises | **27**<br>540 sit-ups<br>540 sitting twists<br>270 leg raises | **28**<br>**200**<br>up and down planks | **29**<br>580 sit-ups<br>580 sitting twists<br>290 leg raises | **30**<br>600 sit-ups<br>600 sitting twists<br>300 leg raises |

# 22    Abs & Core

Strong external abs and a powerful core are the ingredients needed to transform the strength of muscles into power. It takes patience, perseverance and a plan and this 30-day challenge is definitely a good start.

Repeat an exercise of the day 20 times, 4 sets in total with a 20 second rest in between sets. Complete all 30 days.

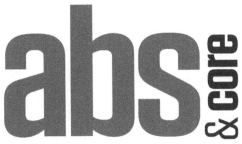

# abs & core

## 30-Day Challenge

20 repetitions each
x 4 sets in total
20 seconds rest between sets

© darebee.com

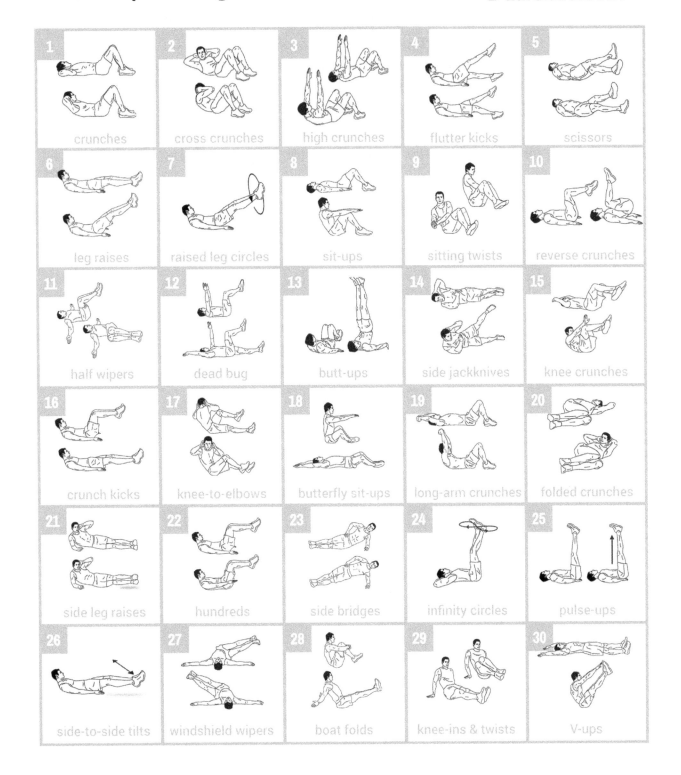

| | | | | |
|---|---|---|---|---|
| **1** crunches | **2** cross crunches | **3** high crunches | **4** flutter kicks | **5** scissors |
| **6** leg raises | **7** raised leg circles | **8** sit-ups | **9** sitting twists | **10** reverse crunches |
| **11** half wipers | **12** dead bug | **13** butt-ups | **14** side jackknives | **15** knee crunches |
| **16** crunch kicks | **17** knee-to-elbows | **18** butterfly sit-ups | **19** long-arm crunches | **20** folded crunches |
| **21** side leg raises | **22** hundreds | **23** side bridges | **24** infinity circles | **25** pulse-ups |
| **26** side-to-side tilts | **27** windshield wipers | **28** boat folds | **29** knee-ins & twists | **30** V-ups |

# 23    Abs Of Steel

Strong abs help you do everything better: you sit, stand, walk, run and jump with greater ease. You are resistant to muscle fatigue. The thing is abs take a lot of work to develop real strength. You are more agile and more powerful. The Abs of Steel 30-day challenge helps you get where you need to be in respect to your abdominal strength by making constant, small gains each day, one day at a time. By the end of the 30-day period you will be able to experience the new, better version of yourself that you will have built.

# abs of steel

## 30-DAY CHALLENGE

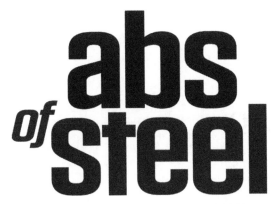
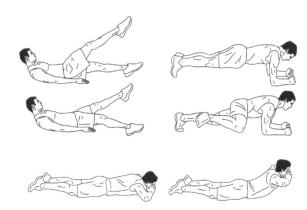

© darebee.com

| | | | | |
|---|---|---|---|---|
| **1**<br>**22** flutter kicks<br>**20sec** rest<br>3 sets | **2**<br>**12** plank crunches<br>**4** back extensions<br>**20sec** rest<br>3 sets | **3**<br>**22** flutter kicks<br>**20sec** rest<br>3 sets | **4**<br>**12** plank crunches<br>**4** back extensions<br>**20sec** rest<br>3 sets | **5**<br>**22** flutter kicks<br>**20sec** rest<br>3 sets |
| **6**<br>**12** plank crunches<br>**4** back extensions<br>**20sec** rest<br>3 sets | **7**<br>**24** flutter kicks<br>**20sec** rest<br>3 sets | **8**<br>**14** plank crunches<br>**4** back extensions<br>**20sec** rest<br>3 sets | **9**<br>**24** flutter kicks<br>**20sec** rest<br>3 sets | **10**<br>**14** plank crunches<br>**4** back extensions<br>**20sec** rest<br>3 sets |
| **11**<br>**24** flutter kicks<br>**20sec** rest<br>3 sets | **12**<br>**14** plank crunches<br>**4** back extensions<br>**20sec** rest<br>3 sets | **13**<br>**26** flutter kicks<br>**20sec** rest<br>3 sets | **14**<br>**16** plank crunches<br>**4** back extensions<br>**20sec** rest<br>3 sets | **15**<br>**26** flutter kicks<br>**20sec** rest<br>3 sets |
| **16**<br>**16** plank crunches<br>**4** back extensions<br>**20sec** rest<br>3 sets | **17**<br>**26** flutter kicks<br>**20sec** rest<br>3 sets | **18**<br>**16** plank crunches<br>**4** back extensions<br>**20sec** rest<br>3 sets | **19**<br>**28** flutter kicks<br>**20sec** rest<br>3 sets | **20**<br>**18** plank crunches<br>**4** back extensions<br>**20sec** rest<br>3 sets |
| **21**<br>**28** flutter kicks<br>**20sec** rest<br>3 sets | **22**<br>**18** plank crunches<br>**4** back extensions<br>**20sec** rest<br>3 sets | **23**<br>**28** flutter kicks<br>**20sec** rest<br>3 sets | **24**<br>**18** plank crunches<br>**4** back extensions<br>**20sec** rest<br>3 sets | **25**<br>**30** flutter kicks<br>**20sec** rest<br>3 sets |
| **26**<br>**20** plank crunches<br>**4** back extensions<br>**20sec** rest<br>3 sets | **27**<br>**30** flutter kicks<br>**20sec** rest<br>3 sets | **28**<br>**20** plank crunches<br>**4** back extensions<br>**20sec** rest<br>3 sets | **29**<br>**30** flutter kicks<br>**20sec** rest<br>3 sets | **30**<br>**20** plank crunches<br>**4** back extensions<br>**20sec** rest<br>3 sets |

## 24 Action Hero

Streamline your body, tighten up your abs and core and strengthen your tendons with the Action Hero Challenge! All heroes have to start somewhere - the hard part is making the first step in the right direction. Once you are on your way it's just working through it, one day at a time, one foot in front of the other. Stick with it for 30 days and you will be ready to jump into action, anytime.

Note: as always, all reps are given in total so 40 side leg raises is 20 reps per leg.

# ACTION HERO

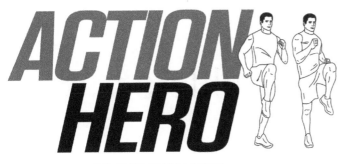
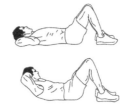
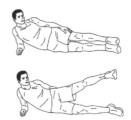

## 30-DAY CHALLENGE

© darebee.com

| | | | | |
|---|---|---|---|---|
| **1**<br>**30** high knees<br>3 sets \| 30sec rest | **2**<br>**15** crunches<br>**30** side leg raises<br>3 sets \| 30sec rest | **3**<br>**30** high knees<br>4 sets \| 30sec rest | **4**<br>**15** crunches<br>**30** side leg raises<br>4 sets \| 30sec rest | **5**<br>**40** high knees<br>3 sets \| 30sec rest |
| **6**<br>**20** crunches<br>**40** side leg raises<br>3 sets \| 30sec rest | **7**<br>**40** high knees<br>4 sets \| 30sec rest | **8**<br>**20** crunches<br>**40** side leg raises<br>4 sets \| 30sec rest | **9**<br>**50** high knees<br>3 sets \| 30sec rest | **10**<br>**25** crunches<br>**50** side leg raises<br>3 sets \| 30sec rest |
| **11**<br>**50** high knees<br>4 sets \| 30sec rest | **12**<br>**25** crunches<br>**50** side leg raises<br>4 sets \| 30sec rest | **13**<br>**60** high knees<br>3 sets \| 30sec rest | **14**<br>**30** crunches<br>**60** side leg raises<br>3 sets \| 30sec rest | **15**<br>**60** high knees<br>4 sets \| 30sec rest |
| **16**<br>**30** crunches<br>**60** side leg raises<br>4 sets \| 30sec rest | **17**<br>**70** high knees<br>3 sets \| 30sec rest | **18**<br>**35** crunches<br>**70** side leg raises<br>3 sets \| 30sec rest | **19**<br>**70** high knees<br>4 sets \| 30sec rest | **20**<br>**35** crunches<br>**70** side leg raises<br>4 sets \| 30sec rest |
| **21**<br>**80** high knees<br>3 sets \| 30sec rest | **22**<br>**40** crunches<br>**80** side leg raises<br>3 sets \| 30sec rest | **23**<br>**80** high knees<br>4 sets \| 30sec rest | **24**<br>**40** crunches<br>**80** side leg raises<br>4 sets \| 30sec rest | **25**<br>**90** high knees<br>3 sets \| 30sec rest |
| **26**<br>**45** crunches<br>**90** side leg raises<br>3 sets \| 30sec rest | **27**<br>**90** high knees<br>4 sets \| 30sec rest | **28**<br>**45** crunches<br>**90** side leg raises<br>4 sets \| 30sec rest | **29**<br>**100** high knees<br>3 sets \| 30sec rest | **30**<br>**50** crunches<br>**100** side leg raises<br>3 sets \| 30sec rest |

## 25 Back & Shoulders

The back and shoulder muscles power a whole range of upper body movements. They help with posture. They play a pivotal part in creating power in physical movement. They allow us to resist fatigue. They are also hard to train. The Back & Shoulders Challenge takes you through a thirty day set of exercises that will completely change your physical awareness of the muscles on your back and shoulders. By the end of it you will have a greater sense of control over these muscles and a deeper connection with your body.

# back & shoulders

## 30-DAY CHALLENGE © darebee.com

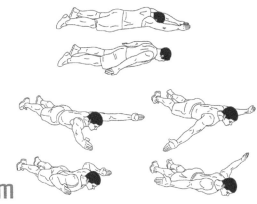

| 1 | 2 | 3 | 4 | 5 |
|---|---|---|---|---|
| **12** reverse angels<br>**30sec** rest<br>3 sets | **6** W-extensions<br>**6** prone reverse flys<br>**30sec** rest<br>3 sets | **12** reverse angels<br>**30sec** rest<br>3 sets | **6** W-extensions<br>**6** prone reverse flys<br>**30sec** rest<br>3 sets | **14** reverse angels<br>**30sec** rest<br>3 sets |
| 6 | 7 | 8 | 9 | 10 |
| **8** W-extensions<br>**8** prone reverse flys<br>**30sec** rest<br>3 sets | **14** reverse angels<br>**30sec** rest<br>3 sets | **8** W-extensions<br>**8** prone reverse flys<br>**30sec** rest<br>3 sets | **16** reverse angels<br>**30sec** rest<br>3 sets | **10** W-extensions<br>**10** prone reverse flys<br>**30sec** rest<br>3 sets |
| 11 | 12 | 13 | 14 | 15 |
| **16** reverse angels<br>**30sec** rest<br>3 sets | **10** W-extensions<br>**10** prone reverse flys<br>**30sec** rest<br>3 sets | **18** reverse angels<br>**30sec** rest<br>3 sets | **12** W-extensions<br>**12** prone reverse flys<br>**30sec** rest<br>3 sets | **18** reverse angels<br>**30sec** rest<br>3 sets |
| 16 | 17 | 18 | 19 | 20 |
| **12** W-extensions<br>**12** prone reverse flys<br>**30sec** rest<br>3 sets | **20** reverse angels<br>**30sec** rest<br>3 sets | **14** W-extensions<br>**14** prone reverse flys<br>**30sec** rest<br>3 sets | **20** reverse angels<br>**30sec** rest<br>3 sets | **14** W-extensions<br>**14** prone reverse flys<br>**30sec** rest<br>3 sets |
| 21 | 22 | 23 | 24 | 25 |
| **22** reverse angels<br>**30sec** rest<br>3 sets | **16** W-extensions<br>**16** prone reverse flys<br>**30sec** rest<br>3 sets | **22** reverse angels<br>**30sec** rest<br>3 sets | **16** W-extensions<br>**16** prone reverse flys<br>**30sec** rest<br>3 sets | **24** reverse angels<br>**30sec** rest<br>3 sets |
| 26 | 27 | 28 | 29 | 30 |
| **18** W-extensions<br>**18** prone reverse flys<br>**30sec** rest<br>3 sets | **24** reverse angels<br>**30sec** rest<br>3 sets | **18** W-extensions<br>**18** prone reverse flys<br>**30sec** rest<br>3 sets | **26** reverse angels<br>**30sec** rest<br>3 sets | **20** W-extensions<br>**20** prone reverse flys<br>**30sec** rest<br>3 sets |

## 26 Balance

A body that knows how to balance makes better use of its own resources when performing physical tasks, can make better use of the space it has around it and is a formidable

Instructions: Balance hold time is a total, change legs halfway through e.g., 4 minutes = 2 minutes per leg. Don't put your leg down during in one go side leg raises.

# balance

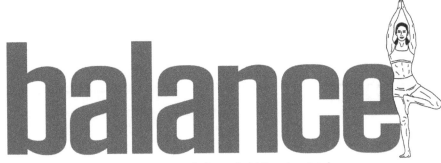
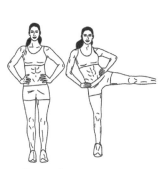

## 30-DAY CHALLENGE

balance hold time is a total,
change legs halfway through

© darebee.com

| | | | | |
|---|---|---|---|---|
| **1** <br> **3 minutes** <br> in one go <br> balance hold | **2** <br> **80** <br> side leg raises <br> throughout the day | **3** <br> **4 minutes** <br> in total <br> balance hold | **4** <br> **80** <br> side leg raises <br> 40/40 in one go | **5** <br> **4 minutes** <br> in one go <br> balance hold |
| **6** <br> **100** <br> side leg raises <br> throughout the day | **7** <br> **5 minutes** <br> in total <br> balance hold | **8** <br> **100** <br> side leg raises <br> 50/50 in one go | **9** <br> **5 minutes** <br> in one go <br> balance hold | **10** <br> **120** <br> side leg raises <br> throughout the day |
| **11** <br> **6 minutes** <br> in total <br> balance hold | **12** <br> **120** <br> side leg raises <br> 60/60 in one go | **13** <br> **6 minutes** <br> in one go <br> balance hold | **14** <br> **140** <br> side leg raises <br> throughout the day | **15** <br> **7 minutes** <br> in total <br> balance hold |
| **16** <br> **140** <br> side leg raises <br> 70/70 in one go | **17** <br> **7 minutes** <br> in one go <br> balance hold | **18** <br> **160** <br> side leg raises <br> throughout the day | **19** <br> **8 minutes** <br> in total <br> balance hold | **20** <br> **160** <br> side leg raises <br> 80/80 in one go |
| **21** <br> **8 minutes** <br> in one go <br> balance hold | **22** <br> **180** <br> side leg raises <br> throughout the day | **23** <br> **9 minutes** <br> in total <br> balance hold | **24** <br> **180** <br> side leg raises <br> 90/90 in one go | **25** <br> **9 minutes** <br> in one go <br> balance hold |
| **26** <br> **200** <br> side leg raises <br> throughout the day | **27** <br> **10 minutes** <br> in total <br> balance hold | **28** <br> **200** <br> side leg raises <br> 100/100 in one go | **29** <br> **10 minutes** <br> in one go <br> balance hold | **30** <br> **2 min** hold <br> followed up by <br> **200** side leg raises |

## 27    Boxer

Combat sports make the greatest fitness demand because of the nature of their competitive element. The body is transformed into a tool where no part of aspect of fitness is overlooked or left to chance. As a result they force us to work on virtually everything. This is why this challenge is so transformative.

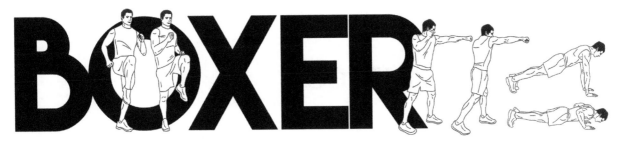

# 30-DAY CHALLENGE

© darebee.com

| | | | | |
|---|---|---|---|---|
| **1**<br>1min high knees<br>1min rest<br>4 sets | **2**<br>10 push-ups<br>40 punches<br>4 sets \| 20sec rest | **3**<br>**400** punches<br>throughout the day | **4**<br>1min non-stop:<br>1 push-up<br>4 punches | **5**<br>20sec high knees<br>20sec punches<br>4 sets \| no rest |
| **6**<br>10 push-ups<br>40 punches<br>4 sets \| no rest | **7**<br>**800** punches<br>throughout the day | **8**<br>1min non-stop:<br>1 push-up<br>4 punches | **9**<br>1min high knees<br>1min rest<br>5 sets | **10**<br>10 push-ups<br>40 punches<br>5 sets \| 20sec rest |
| **11**<br>**1200** punches<br>throughout the day | **12**<br>1min non-stop:<br>1 push-up<br>4 punches | **13**<br>20sec high knees<br>20sec punches<br>5 sets \| no rest | **14**<br>10 push-ups<br>40 punches<br>5 sets \| no rest | **15**<br>**1400** punches<br>throughout the day |
| **16**<br>2min non-stop:<br>1 push-up<br>4 punches | **17**<br>1min high knees<br>1min rest<br>6 sets | **18**<br>10 push-ups<br>40 punches<br>6 sets \| 20sec rest | **19**<br>**1600** punches<br>throughout the day | **20**<br>2min non-stop:<br>1 push-up<br>4 punches |
| **21**<br>20sec high knees<br>20sec punches<br>6 sets \| no rest | **22**<br>10 push-ups<br>40 punches<br>6 sets \| no rest | **23**<br>**1800** punches<br>throughout the day | **24**<br>2min non-stop:<br>1 push-up<br>4 punches | **25**<br>1min high knees<br>1min rest<br>7 sets |
| **26**<br>10 push-ups<br>40 punches<br>7 sets \| 20sec rest | **27**<br>**2000** punches<br>throughout the day | **28**<br>3min non-stop:<br>1 push-up<br>4 punches | **29**<br>20sec high knees<br>20sec punches<br>7 sets \| no rest | **30**<br>10 push-ups<br>40 punches<br>7 sets \| no rest |

## 28 Burpee

Burpees are everyone's favorite gripe and for a good reason. The Burpee Challenge is exactly what you think it is which means that this is a challenge that is mental and physical in equal parts. Your body will do it but only if your mind makes it so. Your mind must change so your body can transform.

# BURPEES

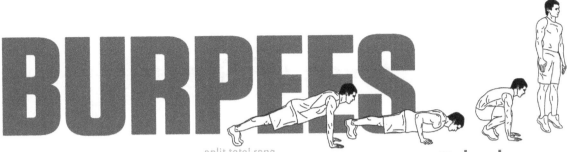

**30-DAY CHALLENGE**  split total reps into manageable sets  © darebee.com

| | | | | |
|---|---|---|---|---|
| **1**<br>**10**<br>burpees | **2**<br>**20**<br>burpees | **3**<br>**25**<br>burpees | **4**<br>30sec plank<br>2 times a day | **5**<br>**25**<br>burpees |
| **6**<br>**30**<br>burpees | **7**<br>**45**<br>burpees | **8**<br>30sec plank<br>3 times a day | **9**<br>**45**<br>burpees | **10**<br>**50**<br>burpees |
| **11**<br>**55**<br>burpees | **12**<br>30sec plank<br>4 times a day | **13**<br>**55**<br>burpees | **14**<br>**60**<br>burpees | **15**<br>**65**<br>burpees |
| **16**<br>45sec plank<br>2 times a day | **17**<br>**65**<br>burpees | **18**<br>**70**<br>burpees | **19**<br>**75**<br>burpees | **20**<br>45sec plank<br>3 times a day |
| **21**<br>**75**<br>burpees | **22**<br>**80**<br>burpees | **23**<br>**85**<br>burpees | **24**<br>45sec plank<br>4 times a day | **25**<br>**85**<br>burpees |
| **26**<br>**90**<br>burpees | **27**<br>**95**<br>burpees | **28**<br>60sec plank<br>5 times a day | **29**<br>**95**<br>burpees | **30**<br>**100**<br>burpees |

## 29 Calves Of Steel

Spartans, Roman Legionnaires, boxers and sprinters have a lot in common when it comes to training their calves. Because they have to squeeze every erg of energy out of the ground force applied when they move, training their calves requires particular focus and dedication. Calves of Steel is a challenge that helps you get, well ... calves of steel.

# calves of steel

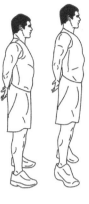

## 30-DAY CHALLENGE
© darebee.com

| | | | | |
|---|---|---|---|---|
| **1**<br>**60** calf raises<br>in total<br>throughout the day | **2**<br>**20 seconds**<br>calf raise hold<br>2 sets \| 30sec rest | **3**<br>**70** calf raises<br>in total<br>throughout the day | **4**<br>**20 seconds**<br>calf raise hold<br>2 sets \| 30sec rest | **5**<br>**80** calf raises<br>in total<br>throughout the day |
| **6**<br>**30 seconds**<br>calf raise hold<br>2 sets \| 30sec rest | **7**<br>**90** calf raises<br>in total<br>throughout the day | **8**<br>**30 seconds**<br>calf raise hold<br>2 sets \| 30sec rest | **9**<br>**100** calf raises<br>in total<br>throughout the day | **10**<br>**40 seconds**<br>calf raise hold<br>2 sets \| 30sec rest |
| **11**<br>**110** calf raises<br>in total<br>throughout the day | **12**<br>**40 seconds**<br>calf raise hold<br>2 sets \| 30sec rest | **13**<br>**120** calf raises<br>in total<br>throughout the day | **14**<br>**50 seconds**<br>calf raise hold<br>2 sets \| 30sec rest | **15**<br>**130** calf raises<br>in total<br>throughout the day |
| **16**<br>**50 seconds**<br>calf raise hold<br>2 sets \| 30sec rest | **17**<br>**140** calf raises<br>in total<br>throughout the day | **18**<br>**60 seconds**<br>calf raise hold<br>2 sets \| 30sec rest | **19**<br>**150** calf raises<br>in total<br>throughout the day | **20**<br>**60 seconds**<br>calf raise hold<br>2 sets \| 30sec rest |
| **21**<br>**160** calf raises<br>in total<br>throughout the day | **22**<br>**1min 10sec**<br>calf raise hold<br>2 sets \| 30sec rest | **23**<br>**170** calf raises<br>in total<br>throughout the day | **24**<br>**1min 10sec**<br>calf raise hold<br>2 sets \| 30sec rest | **25**<br>**180** calf raises<br>in total<br>throughout the day |
| **26**<br>**1min 20sec**<br>calf raise hold<br>2 sets \| 30sec rest | **27**<br>**190** calf raises<br>in total<br>throughout the day | **28**<br>**1min 20sec**<br>calf raise hold<br>2 sets \| 30sec rest | **29**<br>**200** calf raises<br>in total<br>throughout the day | **30**<br>**1min 30sec**<br>calf raise hold<br>2 sets \| 30sec rest |

## 30   Cardio & Abs

Exercises that deliver on more than one aspect of fitness are great time-savers. The Cardio & Abs Challenge will not only test your body but also your discipline as you have to maintain the focus necessary to do the exercises every day, for a month. The result is that key muscle adptations will be triggered that will lead to performance-enhancing results.

# cardio & abs

## 30-DAY CHALLENGE

© darebee.com

| | | | | |
|---|---|---|---|---|
| **1**<br>20 high knees<br>20 climbers<br>3 sets \| 1 min rest | **2**<br>100 flutter kicks<br>in total for the day | **3**<br>1min high knees<br>as fast as you can<br>3 sets \| 1 min rest | **4**<br>1min flutter kicks<br>1 min rest<br>3 sets | **5**<br>20 high knees<br>20 climbers<br>4 sets \| 1 min rest |
| **6**<br>140 flutter kicks<br>in total for the day | **7**<br>1min high knees<br>as fast as you can<br>3 sets \| 1 min rest | **8**<br>1min flutter kicks<br>1 min rest<br>3 sets | **9**<br>30 high knees<br>30 climbers<br>3 sets \| 1 min rest | **10**<br>180 flutter kicks<br>in total for the day |
| **11**<br>1min high knees<br>as fast as you can<br>3 sets \| 1 min rest | **12**<br>1min flutter kicks<br>1 min rest<br>3 sets | **13**<br>30 high knees<br>30 climbers<br>4 sets \| 1 min rest | **14**<br>220 flutter kicks<br>in total for the day | **15**<br>1min high knees<br>as fast as you can<br>3 sets \| 1 min rest |
| **16**<br>1min flutter kicks<br>1 min rest<br>3 sets | **17**<br>40 high knees<br>40 climbers<br>3 sets \| 1 min rest | **18**<br>260 flutter kicks<br>in total for the day | **19**<br>1min high knees<br>as fast as you can<br>3 sets \| 1 min rest | **20**<br>1min flutter kicks<br>1 min rest<br>3 sets |
| **21**<br>40 high knees<br>40 climbers<br>4 sets \| 1 min rest | **22**<br>300 flutter kicks<br>in total for the day | **23**<br>1min high knees<br>as fast as you can<br>3 sets \| 1 min rest | **24**<br>1min flutter kicks<br>1 min rest<br>3 sets | **25**<br>50 high knees<br>50 climbers<br>3 sets \| 1 min rest |
| **26**<br>340 flutter kicks<br>in total for the day | **27**<br>1min high knees<br>as fast as you can<br>3 sets \| 1 min rest | **28**<br>1min flutter kicks<br>1 min rest<br>3 sets | **29**<br>50 high knees<br>50 climbers<br>4 sets \| 1 min rest | **30**<br>400 flutter kicks<br>in total for the day |

## 31 Cardio Blast

Just one session of cardio-based physical activity has deep neurochemical and neurobiological effects on the body. In this challenge, over 30 days, you get the chance to change your body and mind at a deep, fundamental level that will help you level up. Cardio Blast is as much a mental challenge then as it is a physical one.

# CARDIO BLAST

**30-DAY CHALLENGE**

split total reps into manageable sets

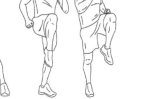

© darebee.com

| | | | | |
|---|---|---|---|---|
| **1** 50 jumping jacks | **2** 60 high knees | **3** 100 jumping jacks | **4** 80 high knees | **5** 150 jumping jacks |
| **6** 100 high knees | **7** 200 jumping jacks | **8** 120 high knees | **9** 250 jumping jacks | **10** 140 high knees |
| **11** 300 jumping jacks | **12** 160 high knees | **13** 350 jumping jacks | **14** 180 high knees | **15** 400 jumping jacks |
| **16** 200 high knees | **17** 450 jumping jacks | **18** 220 high knees | **19** 500 jumping jacks | **20** 240 high knees |
| **21** 550 jumping jacks | **22** 260 high knees | **23** 600 jumping jacks | **24** 280 high knees | **25** 650 jumping jacks |
| **26** 300 high knees | **27** 700 jumping jacks | **28** 320 high knees | **29** 750 jumping jacks | **30** 340 high knees |

# 32 Cardio

Developing good cardiovascular fitness helps fight fatigue, unlocks mental focus and helps keep muscles, lungs and heart functioning at peak performance levels. The Cardio Challenge is key to helpiing you meet your fitness goals on all these attributes of physical fitness and mental and psychologicall wellbeing.

# cardio

## 30-DAY CHALLENGE

split total reps into manageable sets

© darebee.com

| 1 | 2 | 3 | 4 | 5 |
|---|---|---|---|---|
| 40 high knees<br>20 climbers | 60 high knees<br>40 climbers | 20 high knees<br>60 climbers | 40 high knees<br>20 climbers | 60 high knees<br>40 climbers |

| 6 | 7 | 8 | 9 | 10 |
|---|---|---|---|---|
| 60 high knees<br>20 climbers | 80 high knees<br>40 climbers | 40 high knees<br>20 climbers | 80 high knees<br>40 climbers | 80 high knees<br>60 climbers |

| 11 | 12 | 13 | 14 | 15 |
|---|---|---|---|---|
| 100 high knees<br>20 climbers | 80 high knees<br>40 climbers | 40 high knees<br>40 climbers | 80 high knees<br>60 climbers | 100 high knees<br>60 climbers |

| 16 | 17 | 18 | 19 | 20 |
|---|---|---|---|---|
| 140 high knees<br>40 climbers | 100 high knees<br>40 climbers | 40 high knees<br>80 climbers | 100 high knees<br>40 climbers | 140 high knees<br>60 climbers |

| 21 | 22 | 23 | 24 | 25 |
|---|---|---|---|---|
| 160 high knees<br>40 climbers | 120 high knees<br>60 climbers | 60 high knees<br>20 climbers | 100 high knees<br>40 climbers | 160 high knees<br>20 climbers |

| 26 | 27 | 28 | 29 | 30 |
|---|---|---|---|---|
| 200 high knees<br>20 climbers | 160 high knees<br>40 climbers | 100 high knees<br>20 climbers | 100 high knees<br>80 climbers | 240 high knees<br>60 climbers |

## 33 Cardio HIIT

Technically all High Intensity Interval Training (HIIT) exercises have a strong component of cardio training. To produce an HIIT Challenge that specifically focuses on cardio fitness however takes the whole thing up one level which is why this is a challenge you must conquer if you want to increase your cardiovascular health.

# cardio HIIT

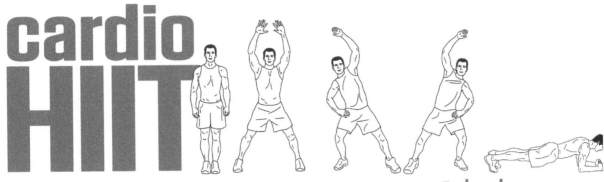

## 30-DAY CHALLENGE

© darebee.com

| 1 | 2 | 3 | 4 | 5 |
|---|---|---|---|---|
| **30sec** side jack<br>**30sec** jumping jacks<br>6 sets \| **1min** rest | **30sec** elbow plank<br>2 sets \| 30sec rest | **30sec** side jack<br>**30sec** jumping jacks<br>6 sets \| **1min** rest | **30sec** elbow plank<br>2 sets \| 30sec rest | **30sec** side jack<br>**30sec** jumping jacks<br>6 sets \| **1min** rest |
| **6** | **7** | **8** | **9** | **10** |
| **30sec** elbow plank<br>2 sets \| 30sec rest | **30sec** side jack<br>**30sec** jumping jacks<br>7 sets \| **1min** rest | **30sec** elbow plank<br>3 sets \| 30sec rest | **30sec** side jack<br>**30sec** jumping jacks<br>7 sets \| **1min** rest | **30sec** elbow plank<br>3 sets \| 30sec rest |
| **11** | **12** | **13** | **14** | **15** |
| **30sec** side jack<br>**30sec** jumping jacks<br>7 sets \| **1min** rest | **30sec** elbow plank<br>3 sets \| 30sec rest | **30sec** side jack<br>**30sec** jumping jacks<br>8 sets \| **1min** rest | **30sec** elbow plank<br>4 sets \| 30sec rest | **30sec** side jack<br>**30sec** jumping jacks<br>8 sets \| **1min** rest |
| **16** | **17** | **18** | **19** | **20** |
| **30sec** elbow plank<br>4 sets \| 30sec rest | **30sec** side jack<br>**30sec** jumping jacks<br>8 sets \| **1min** rest | **30sec** elbow plank<br>4 sets \| 30sec rest | **30sec** side jack<br>**30sec** jumping jacks<br>9 sets \| **1min** rest | **30sec** elbow plank<br>5 sets \| 30sec rest |
| **21** | **22** | **23** | **24** | **25** |
| **30sec** side jack<br>**30sec** jumping jacks<br>9 sets \| **1min** rest | **30sec** elbow plank<br>5 sets \| 30sec rest | **30sec** side jack<br>**30sec** jumping jacks<br>9 sets \| **1min** rest | **30sec** elbow plank<br>5 sets \| 30sec rest | **30sec** side jack<br>**30sec** jumping jacks<br>10 sets \| **1min** rest |
| **26** | **27** | **28** | **29** | **30** |
| **30sec** elbow plank<br>6 sets \| 30sec rest | **30sec** side jack<br>**30sec** jumping jacks<br>10 sets \| **1min** rest | **30sec** elbow plank<br>6 sets \| 30sec rest | **30sec** side jack<br>**30sec** jumping jacks<br>10 sets \| **1min** rest | **30sec** elbow plank<br>6 sets \| 30sec rest |

## 34   Chest & Arms

Chisel your arms and pump up your chest with this 30-day challenge! Get extra definition in your upperbody and lift your pecs. It's perfect for men and especially good for women (a sports bra is highly recommended for this challenge). The challenge works primarily your chest, triceps, abs and core.

Push-ups "to failure" stands for your maximum, do as many repetitions as you can whether it's 4 push-ups or 40 - just do your best every time. It's ok to substitute with knee push-ups if a full push-up is not something you can do yet.

Tip: if you own a pair of dumbbells you can do renegade rows instead of shoulder taps for additional back and biceps work. If your dumbbells are over 8kg (16lb) halve the number of reps per set.

# chest & arms

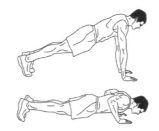
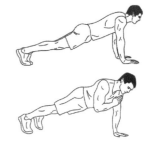

## 30-DAY CHALLENGE

© darebee.com

| | | | | |
|---|---|---|---|---|
| **1**<br>**to failure**<br>push-ups<br>3 sets \| 30sec rest | **2**<br>**20** shoulder taps<br>3 sets \| 30sec rest | **3**<br>**to failure**<br>push-ups<br>3 sets \| 30sec rest | **4**<br>**22** shoulder taps<br>3 sets \| 30sec rest | **5**<br>**to failure**<br>push-ups<br>3 sets \| 30sec rest |
| **6**<br>**24** shoulder taps<br>3 sets \| 30sec rest | **7**<br>**to failure**<br>push-ups<br>3 sets \| 30sec rest | **8**<br>**20** shoulder taps<br>4 sets \| 30sec rest | **9**<br>**to failure**<br>push-ups<br>3 sets \| 30sec rest | **10**<br>**22** shoulder taps<br>4 sets \| 30sec rest |
| **11**<br>**to failure**<br>push-ups<br>4 sets \| 30sec rest | **12**<br>**24** shoulder taps<br>4 sets \| 30sec rest | **13**<br>**to failure**<br>push-ups<br>4 sets \| 30sec rest | **14**<br>**20** shoulder taps<br>5 sets \| 30sec rest | **15**<br>**to failure**<br>push-ups<br>4 sets \| 30sec rest |
| **16**<br>**22** shoulder taps<br>5 sets \| 30sec rest | **17**<br>**to failure**<br>push-ups<br>4 sets \| 30sec rest | **18**<br>**24** shoulder taps<br>5 sets \| 30sec rest | **19**<br>**to failure**<br>push-ups<br>4 sets \| 30sec rest | **20**<br>**20** shoulder taps<br>6 sets \| 30sec rest |
| **21**<br>**to failure**<br>push-ups<br>5 sets \| 30sec rest | **22**<br>**22** shoulder taps<br>6 sets \| 30sec rest | **23**<br>**to failure**<br>push-ups<br>5 sets \| 30sec rest | **24**<br>**24** shoulder taps<br>6 sets \| 30sec rest | **25**<br>**to failure**<br>push-ups<br>5 sets \| 30sec rest |
| **26**<br>**20** shoulder taps<br>7 sets \| 30sec rest | **27**<br>**to failure**<br>push-ups<br>5 sets \| 30sec rest | **28**<br>**22** shoulder taps<br>7 sets \| 30sec rest | **29**<br>**to failure**<br>push-ups<br>5 sets \| 30sec rest | **30**<br>**24** shoulder taps<br>7 sets \| 30sec rest |

## 35   Core

Training the transverse abdominis muscle (also known as the core) helps maintain posture, balance, stability and may help in the health of the internal organs that are in the lower abdominal region. This is a challenge that will create the basis you need for a strong and stable core.

# core

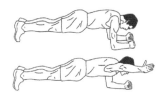

**30-DAY CHALLENGE**  split total reps into manageable sets

© darebee.com

| 1 | 2 | 3 | 4 | 5 |
|---|---|---|---|---|
| 6 push-ups<br>15 second plank<br>10 plank reaches | 10 push-ups<br>15 second plank<br>12 plank reaches | 12 push-ups<br>15 second plank<br>14 plank reaches | 60 second plank<br>10 plank reaches | 14 push-ups<br>15 second plank<br>16 plank reaches |
| **6** | **7** | **8** | **9** | **10** |
| 16 push-ups<br>20 second plank<br>18 plank reaches | 20 push-ups<br>20 second plank<br>20 plank reaches | 60 second plank<br>10 plank reaches | 22 push-ups<br>20 second plank<br>22 plank reaches | 24 push-ups<br>20 second plank<br>24 plank reaches |
| **11** | **12** | **13** | **14** | **15** |
| 26 push-ups<br>25 second plank<br>26 plank reaches | 60 second plank<br>10 plank reaches | 28 push-ups<br>25 second plank<br>28 plank reaches | 30 push-ups<br>25 second plank<br>30 plank reaches | 32 push-ups<br>25 second plank<br>32 plank reaches |
| **16** | **17** | **18** | **19** | **20** |
| 60 second plank<br>10 plank reaches | 34 push-ups<br>30 second plank<br>34 plank reaches | 36 push-ups<br>30 second plank<br>36 plank reaches | 38 push-ups<br>30 second plank<br>38 plank reaches | 60 second plank<br>10 plank reaches |
| **21** | **22** | **23** | **24** | **25** |
| 40 push-ups<br>35 second plank<br>40 plank reaches | 42 push-ups<br>35 second plank<br>42 plank reaches | 46 push-ups<br>35 second plank<br>44 plank reaches | 60 second plank<br>10 plank reaches | 48 push-ups<br>35 second plank<br>46 plank reaches |
| **26** | **27** | **28** | **29** | **30** |
| 50 push-ups<br>40 second plank<br>48 plank reaches | 52 push-ups<br>40 second plank<br>50 plank reaches | 60 second plank<br>10 plank reaches | 54 push-ups<br>45 second plank<br>52 plank reaches | 60 push-ups<br>45 second plank<br>60 plank reaches |

## 36     Core Control

Core strength is important in helping the body fight fatigue, prevent injury from overload and power explosiveness. A strong core preserves momentum as muscles transfer power from the upper body to the lower body (when running or sprinting, for instance) and the lower body to the upper body (like when punching). A strong core then helps develop physical power by minimizing the loss of force transfer across the body's muscles. Core Control will help you develop your core. As you feel yourself getting stronger you will find yourself becoming more physically capable.

Split total reps into manageable sets.

# core control

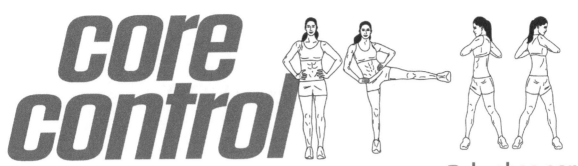

## 30-DAY CHALLENGE

© darebee.com

| | | | | |
|---|---|---|---|---|
| **1**<br>**40**<br>torso twists | **2**<br>**60**<br>side leg raises | **3**<br>**40**<br>torso twists | **4**<br>**70**<br>side leg raises | **5**<br>**40**<br>torso twists |
| **6**<br>**80**<br>side leg raises | **7**<br>**40**<br>torso twists | **8**<br>**90**<br>side leg raises | **9**<br>**40**<br>torso twists | **10**<br>**100**<br>side leg raises |
| **11**<br>**40**<br>torso twists | **12**<br>**110**<br>side leg raises | **13**<br>**40**<br>torso twists | **14**<br>**120**<br>side leg raises | **15**<br>**40**<br>torso twists |
| **16**<br>**130**<br>side leg raises | **17**<br>**40**<br>torso twists | **18**<br>**140**<br>side leg raises | **19**<br>**40**<br>torso twists | **20**<br>**150**<br>side leg raises |
| **21**<br>**40**<br>torso twists | **22**<br>**160**<br>side leg raises | **23**<br>**40**<br>torso twists | **24**<br>**170**<br>side leg raises | **25**<br>**40**<br>torso twists |
| **26**<br>**180**<br>side leg raises | **27**<br>**40**<br>torso twists | **28**<br>**190**<br>side leg raises | **29**<br>**40**<br>torso twists | **30**<br>**200**<br>side leg raises |

## 37 Daily Gratitude

Neuroscientific studies have demonstrated that at the brain level, neural mechanisms involved in moral judgments and feelings of gratefulness are evoked in the right anterior temporal cortex of the brain. In the same studies, it was revealed that the reason why some of us are naturally more grateful than others, is down to neurochemical differences at the Central Nervous System. People who express and feel gratitude have a higher volume of grey matter in the right inferior temporal gyrus. This is an area of the brain that is involved in a number of cognitive processes, including semantic memory processing, language processes, visual perception, and the integration of information from different senses.

When we express gratitude and receive the same, our brain releases dopamine and serotonin, the two crucial neurotransmitters responsible for our emotions, and they make us feel 'good'. They enhance our mood immediately, making us feel happy from the inside. By consciously practicing gratitude everyday, we can help these neural pathways to strengthen themselves and ultimately create a permanent grateful and positive nature within ourselves that affects everything, from how we perceive the world to how we see ourselves and our capabilities.

The Daily Gratitude Challenge is designed to help you achieve a better state of inner and outer being through the rewiring of your brain's neural pathways.

Instructions: Sit down in a quite place, relax, take a deep breath and mentally list three things you are grateful for today. Repeat the same exercise every day for 30 days. If you can, say the three things aloud. You are not limited by three things but three is the minimum. The list can vary or stay the same from day to day.

When we express gratitude and receive the same, our brain releases dopamine and serotonin, the two crucial neurotransmitters responsible for our emotions, and they make us feel 'good'. They enhance our mood immediately, making us feel happy from the inside. By consciously practicing gratitude everyday, we can help these neural pathways to strengthen themselves and ultimately create a permanent grateful and positive nature within ourselves that affects everything, from how we perceive the world to how we see ourselves and our capabilities.

The Daily Gratitude Challenge is designed to help you achieve a better state of inner and outer being through the rewiring of your brain's neural pathways.

Instructions: Sit down in a quite place, relax, take a deep breath and mentally list three things you are grateful for today. Repeat the same exercise every day for 30 days. If you can, say the three things aloud. You are not limited by three things but three is the minimum. The list can vary or stay the same from day to day.

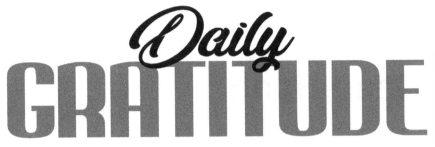

# Daily GRATITUDE

## 30-DAY CHALLENGE

Name three things you are grateful for every day for 30 days.

Ⓒ darebee.com

| | | | | |
|---|---|---|---|---|
| **1** Done! | **2** Done! | **3** Done! | **4** Done! | **5** Done! |
| **6** Done! | **7** Done! | **8** Done! | **9** Done! | **10** Done! |
| **11** Done! | **12** Done! | **13** Done! | **14** Done! | **15** Done! |
| **16** Done! | **17** Done! | **18** Done! | **19** Done! | **20** Done! |
| **21** Done! | **22** Done! | **23** Done! | **24** Done! | **25** Done! |
| **26** Done! | **27** Done! | **28** Done! | **29** Done! | **30** Done! |

## 38 Dead Hang

No exercise is more deceptive than the dead hang and never has just "hanging around" being a harder thing to do. There are multiple benefits that will be gained from this exercise: Improved grip strength, fascial fitness, stronger upper back, improved shoulder strength, improved posture, core fitness and abs. The list of muscles involved alone hints at why what looks so easy is actually such a hard thing to do. The Dead Hang Challenge is designed to help you improve all of this. It will really make you stronger and you will feel and look fitter. Follow the daily guidelines.

Get though the hang time required each day and if there is some day when your grip is not yet strong enough, hold on as long as you can. The moment it fails hang again, immediately and make up the time.

# DEAD HANG
## 30-DAY CHALLENGE

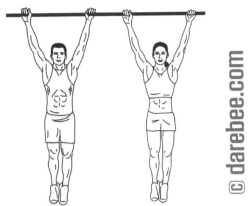

© darebee.com

| 1 | 2 | 3 | 4 | 5 |
|---|---|---|---|---|
| **10 seconds** 2 sets 30 seconds rest | **20 seconds** | **10 seconds** 2 sets 30 seconds rest | **25 seconds** | **10 seconds** 2 sets 30 seconds rest |
| 6 | 7 | 8 | 9 | 10 |
| **30 seconds** | **10 seconds** 2 sets 30 seconds rest | **35 seconds** | **10 seconds** 2 sets 30 seconds rest | **40 seconds** |
| 11 | 12 | 13 | 14 | 15 |
| **10 seconds** 2 sets 30 seconds rest | **45 seconds** | **10 seconds** 2 sets 30 seconds rest | **50 seconds** | **10 seconds** 2 sets 30 seconds rest |
| 16 | 17 | 18 | 19 | 20 |
| **55 seconds** | **10 seconds** 2 sets 30 seconds rest | **60 seconds** | **10 seconds** 2 sets 30 seconds rest | **1min 10sec** |
| 21 | 22 | 23 | 24 | 25 |
| **10 seconds** 2 sets 30 seconds rest | **1min 20sec** | **10 seconds** 2 sets 30 seconds rest | **1min 30sec** | **10 seconds** 2 sets 30 seconds rest |
| 26 | 27 | 28 | 29 | 30 |
| **1min 40sec** | **10 seconds** 2 sets 30 seconds rest | **1min 50sec** | **10 seconds** 2 sets 30 seconds rest | **2 minutes** |

## 39 De-Stress

Nothing gets rid of stress faster than throwing punches. They move your whole body. They engage many complex centers of your brain. It is a physical exercise with a high level of cognitive activation. This 30-day challenge will help you get rid of stress, get fitter, move in a much slicker way and develop the kind of high-level physical awareness enjoyed by those who train their body for combat.

# de-stress

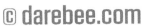

## 30-DAY CHALLENGE

© darebee.com

| | | | | |
|---|---|---|---|---|
| **1**<br>**100**<br>punches | **2**<br>**100**<br>punches | **3**<br>**100**<br>punches | **4**<br>**100**<br>punches | **5**<br>**100**<br>punches |
| **6**<br>**100**<br>punches | **7**<br>**100**<br>punches | **8**<br>**100**<br>punches | **9**<br>**100**<br>punches | **10**<br>**100**<br>punches |
| **11**<br>**100**<br>punches | **12**<br>**100**<br>punches | **13**<br>**100**<br>punches | **14**<br>**100**<br>punches | **15**<br>**100**<br>punches |
| **16**<br>**100**<br>punches | **17**<br>**100**<br>punches | **18**<br>**100**<br>punches | **19**<br>**100**<br>punches | **20**<br>**100**<br>punches |
| **21**<br>**100**<br>punches | **22**<br>**100**<br>punches | **23**<br>**100**<br>punches | **24**<br>**100**<br>punches | **25**<br>**100**<br>punches |
| **26**<br>**100**<br>punches | **27**<br>**100**<br>punches | **28**<br>**100**<br>punches | **29**<br>**100**<br>punches | **30**<br>**100**<br>punches |

## 40 Endurance

Endure the exercises for the given amount of time, don't stop! You can lower the intensity of high knees (don't bring your knees as high) as you tire out but keep on moving. If you drop the plank, pick it back up as soon as you can and continue. Even if you pause or stop, start again as soon as possible keeping the break to the absolute minimum. Earn the extra credit for this challenge: no breaks, no pauses throughout.

# endurance

## 30-day challenge

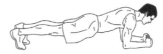

© darebee.com

| | | | | |
|---|---|---|---|---|
| **1**<br>**1 minute**<br>high knees<br>non-stop | **2**<br>**30 seconds**<br>elbow plank<br>in one go | **3**<br>**1min 30sec**<br>high knees<br>non-stop | **4**<br>**40 seconds**<br>elbow plank<br>in one go | **5**<br>**2 minutes**<br>high knees<br>non-stop |
| **6**<br>**60 seconds**<br>elbow plank<br>in one go | **7**<br>**2min 30sec**<br>high knees<br>non-stop | **8**<br>**1min 20sec**<br>elbow plank<br>in one go | **9**<br>**3 minutes**<br>high knees<br>non-stop | **10**<br>**1min 40sec**<br>elbow plank<br>in one go |
| **11**<br>**3min 30sec**<br>high knees<br>non-stop | **12**<br>**2 minutes**<br>elbow plank<br>in one go | **13**<br>**4 minutes**<br>high knees<br>non-stop | **14**<br>**2min 20sec**<br>elbow plank<br>in one go | **15**<br>**4min 30sec**<br>high knees<br>non-stop |
| **16**<br>**2min 40sec**<br>elbow plank<br>in one go | **17**<br>**5 minutes**<br>high knees<br>non-stop | **18**<br>**3 minutes**<br>elbow plank<br>in one go | **19**<br>**5min 30sec**<br>high knees<br>non-stop | **20**<br>**3min 20sec**<br>elbow plank<br>in one go |
| **21**<br>**6 minutes**<br>high knees<br>non-stop | **22**<br>**3min 40sec**<br>elbow plank<br>in one go | **23**<br>**6min 30sec**<br>high knees<br>non-stop | **24**<br>**4 minutes**<br>elbow plank<br>in one go | **25**<br>**7 minutes**<br>high knees<br>non-stop |
| **26**<br>**4min 20sec**<br>elbow plank<br>in one go | **27**<br>**7min 30sec**<br>high knees<br>non-stop | **28**<br>**4min 40sec**<br>elbow plank<br>in one go | **29**<br>**8 minutes**<br>high knees<br>non-stop | **30**<br>**5 minutes**<br>elbow plank<br>in one go |

## 41 Everest

Mountains are here to be climbed and Challenges are here to be conquered. Climbers activate muscle groups throughout the body, they work the core and are great for strengthening tendons and ligaments and increasing functional strength.

Climb the Mount Everest (8,848m) in 30 days! Split total reps into manageable sets throughout the day. All reps are given in total so left + right legs = 2 climbers.

# EVEREST

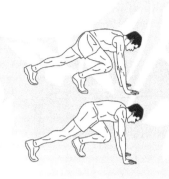

DAREBEE CHALLENGE - climb **8,848m** in 30 days   © darebee.com

| | | | | |
|---|---|---|---|---|
| **1** 60 climbers | **2** 220 climbers | **3** 60 climbers | **4** 240 climbers | **5** 60 climbers |
| **6** 280 climbers | **7** 60 climbers | **8** 320 climbers | **9** 60 climbers | **10** 420 climbers |
| **11** 60 climbers | **12** 460 climbers | **13** 60 climbers | **14** 520 climbers | **15** 60 climbers |
| **16** 540 climbers | **17** 60 climbers | **18** 580 climbers | **19** 60 climbers | **20** 620 climbers |
| **21** 60 climbers | **22** 680 climbers | **23** 60 climbers | **24** 720 climbers | **25** 60 climbers |
| **26** 760 climbers | **27** 60 climbers | **28** 780 climbers | **29** 60 climbers | **30** 808 climbers |

## 42 Fiber

Up your fiber intake: hit the 30g mark every day for 30 days to improve your overall health and digestion. In the process of completing the challenge you will learn more about high fiber foods and what they are and develop a habit of adding them to your menu without even thinking about it. You may be surprised how little fiber you ate before and how good you will feel once you rectify the situation.

# Fiber 30

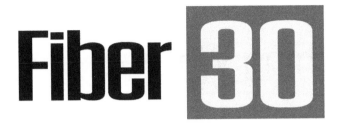

**Eat 30g of fiber a day
for 30 days**
© darebee.com

| | | | | |
|---|---|---|---|---|
| **1** Hit the target today! | **2** Hit the target today! | **3** Hit the target today! | **4** Hit the target today! | **5** Hit the target today! |
| **6** Hit the target today! | **7** Hit the target today! | **8** Hit the target today! | **9** Hit the target today! | **10** Hit the target today! |
| **11** Hit the target today! | **12** Hit the target today! | **13** Hit the target today! | **14** Hit the target today! | **15** Hit the target today! |
| **16** Hit the target today! | **17** Hit the target today! | **18** Hit the target today! | **19** Hit the target today! | **20** Hit the target today! |
| **21** Hit the target today! | **22** Hit the target today! | **23** Hit the target today! | **24** Hit the target today! | **25** Hit the target today! |
| **26** Hit the target today! | **27** Hit the target today! | **28** Hit the target today! | **29** Hit the target today! | **30** Hit the target today! |

## 43 First Thing Water

Drink a glass of water on an empty stomach first thing after you wake up, every day for 30 days. Simple. But there is a lot more to it than that. Water is absorbed by the body much faster than any other fluid and although some of it is processed by and stored in the small intestine at a much slower rate in order to avoid overflooding the blood with fluid, that first jolt of water in the morning helps stabilize blood fluid volume and kick-start a whole lot of other beneficial processes.

# FIRST THING WATER

## 30-DAY CHALLENGE

© darebee.com

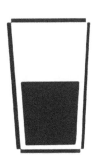

DRINK A GLASS OF WATER RIGHT AFTER WAKING UP

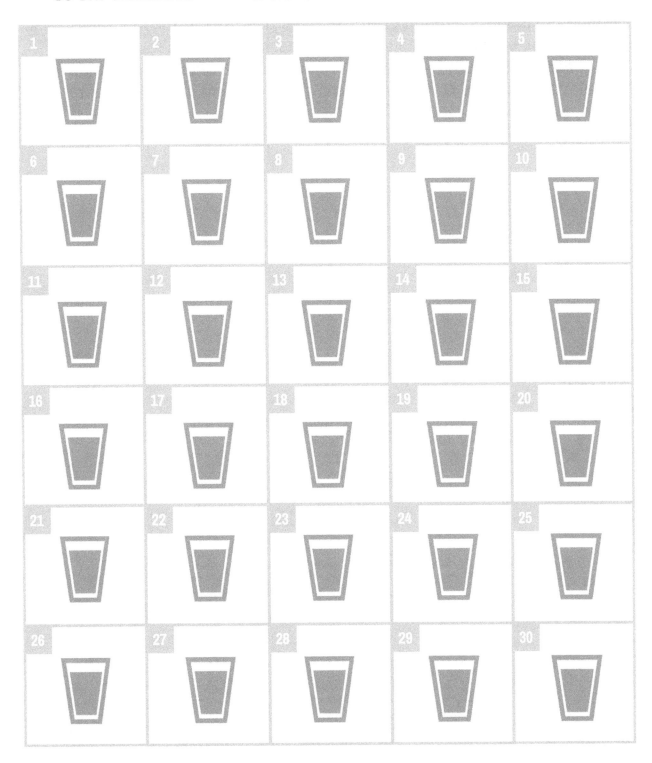

## 44     Five Minute Plank

Holding the plank is a tough exercise. It recruits the rectus abdominis (also known as the core abs) but it also activates, hip flexors, shoulders, pecs and quads. This is why building up to a five minute plank hold is a target well worth aiming for. Its benefits extend well beyond just strong abs.

# FIVE MINUTE PLANK

## 30-DAY CHALLENGE

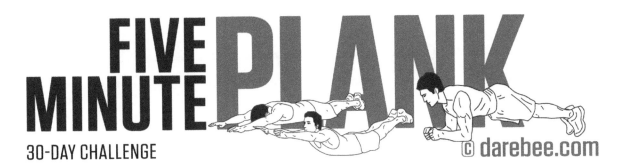

© darebee.com

| 1 | 2 | 3 | 4 | 5 |
|---|---|---|---|---|
| 20 seconds elbow plank | 25 seconds elbow plank | 30 seconds elbow plank | 10 reps supermen 2 sets in total any rest | 45 seconds elbow plank |
| **6** | **7** | **8** | **9** | **10** |
| 60 seconds elbow plank | 1min 10sec elbow plank | 12 reps supermen 2 sets in total any rest | 1min 30sec elbow plank | 1min 40sec elbow plank |
| **11** | **12** | **13** | **14** | **15** |
| 1min 45sec elbow plank | 15 reps supermen 2 sets in total any rest | 2 minute elbow plank | 2min 10sec elbow plank | 2min 30sec elbow plank |
| **16** | **17** | **18** | **19** | **20** |
| 2min 40sec elbow plank | 16 reps supermen 2 sets in total any rest | 3 minute elbow plank | 3min 20sec elbow plank | 3min 30sec elbow plank |
| **21** | **22** | **23** | **24** | **25** |
| 18 reps supermen 2 sets in total any rest | 3min 40sec elbow plank | 3min 50sec elbow plank | 4 minute elbow plank | 4min 20sec elbow plank |
| **26** | **27** | **28** | **29** | **30** |
| 20 reps supermen 2 sets in total any rest | 4min 30sec elbow plank | 4min 40sec elbow plank | 25 reps supermen 2 sets in total any rest | 5 minute elbow plank |

# 45 Flexibility

Lower body flexibility increases the range of motion of joints and enables muscles to move with much lower resistance. This helps deliver fluidity of movement and increased physical power. It also helps reduce fatigue during exercise by making the muscles more supple, cuts down on the incidence of injury and helps achieve greater physical control of the body.

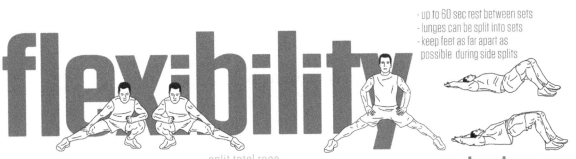

# flexibility

## 30-DAY CHALLENGE

split total reps into manageable sets

- up to 60 sec rest between sets
- lunges can be split into sets
- keep feet as far apart as possible during side splits

© darebee.com

| 1 | 2 | 3 | 4 | 5 |
|---|---|---|---|---|
| 40 side lunges<br>30sec side splits | 40 side lunges<br>35sec side splits | 40 side lunges<br>40sec side splits | 10 bridges<br>3 sets in total | 60 side lunges<br>45sec side splits |

| 6 | 7 | 8 | 9 | 10 |
|---|---|---|---|---|
| 60 side lunges<br>50sec side splits | 60 side lunges<br>55sec side splits | 10 bridges<br>4 sets in total | 80 side lunges<br>1min side splits | 80 side lunges<br>1m10s side splits |

| 11 | 12 | 13 | 14 | 15 |
|---|---|---|---|---|
| 80 side lunges<br>1m20s side splits | 10 bridges<br>5 sets in total | 100 side lunges<br>1m30s side splits | 100 side lunges<br>1m40s side splits | 100 side lunges<br>2min side splits |

| 16 | 17 | 18 | 19 | 20 |
|---|---|---|---|---|
| 20 bridges<br>3 sets in total | 120 side lunges<br>2m10s side splits | 120 side lunges<br>2m20s side splits | 120 side lunges<br>2m30s side splits | 20 bridges<br>4 sets in total |

| 21 | 22 | 23 | 24 | 25 |
|---|---|---|---|---|
| 140 side lunges<br>2m40s side splits | 140 side lunges<br>2m50s side splits | 140 side lunges<br>3min side splits | 20 bridges<br>5 sets in total | 160 side lunges<br>3m10s side splits |

| 26 | 27 | 28 | 29 | 30 |
|---|---|---|---|---|
| 160 side lunges<br>3m20s side splits | 160 side lunges<br>3m40s side splits | 25 bridges<br>4 sets in total | 180 side lunges<br>3m40s side splits | 200 side lunges<br>4min side splits |

## 46 Flex Hang

The flexed arm is a great demonstration of impressive strength to bodyweight ratio and is often used as a measure of upper body endurance. The United States Marine Corps uses it as a physical test with Marines required to take it (and pass it) twice a year. The minimum time they must hold in order to pass is 15 seconds and the maximum they are expected to hold in order to get a flying pass is 70 seconds. This suggests the level of difficulty of the exercise. Upper body strength improves gradually, with time and persistence. The Flex Hang Challenge will help you get stronger and will improve your overall level of fitness by increasing strength across several important, upper body muscle groups. Once you get through the challenge, like the U.S. Marines, you should aim to test yourself at least twice a year and work on workouts that help improve upper body strength; throughout the year.

Split the total amount required into manageable sets, when necessary.

# FLEX HANG
## 30-DAY CHALLENGE

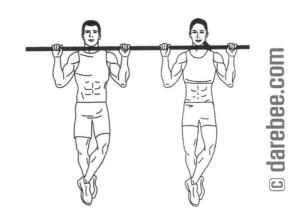

© darebee.com

| 1 | 2 | 3 | 4 | 5 |
|---|---|---|---|---|
| **5 seconds**<br>3 sets<br>30 seconds rest | **10 seconds** | **5 seconds**<br>3 sets<br>30 seconds rest | **10 seconds** | **5 seconds**<br>3 sets<br>30 seconds rest |
| **6** | **7** | **8** | **9** | **10** |
| **15 seconds** | **5 seconds**<br>3 sets<br>30 seconds rest | **15 seconds** | **5 seconds**<br>3 sets<br>30 seconds rest | **20 seconds** |
| **11** | **12** | **13** | **14** | **15** |
| **5 seconds**<br>3 sets<br>30 seconds rest | **20 seconds** | **5 seconds**<br>3 sets<br>30 seconds rest | **25 seconds** | **5 seconds**<br>3 sets<br>30 seconds rest |
| **16** | **17** | **18** | **19** | **20** |
| **25 seconds** | **5 seconds**<br>3 sets<br>30 seconds rest | **30 seconds** | **5 seconds**<br>3 sets<br>30 seconds rest | **30 seconds** |
| **21** | **22** | **23** | **24** | **25** |
| **5 seconds**<br>3 sets<br>30 seconds rest | **35 seconds** | **5 seconds**<br>3 sets<br>30 seconds rest | **35 seconds** | **5 seconds**<br>3 sets<br>30 seconds rest |
| **26** | **27** | **28** | **29** | **30** |
| **40 seconds** | **5 seconds**<br>3 sets<br>30 seconds rest | **40 seconds** | **5 seconds**<br>3 sets<br>30 seconds rest | **45 seconds** |

## 47 Get To Bed On Time

Science tells us that sleep is important for brain health. It is also the time the body uses to repair itself and build muscle. Yet our civilization suffers from a sleep deficit. Life, work and fun conspire to get in the way, creating a 24-hour lifestyle that takes its toll on our physical, mental and psychological health. The Get To Bed Challenge redresses the balance. Aim to get to bed on time, for a month. Feel the difference that will make to your overall sense of wellbeing.

# Get To Bed on time

Pick a time by which you should be in bed every day and stick to it for 30 days in a row

© darebee.com

| | | | | |
|---|---|---|---|---|
| **1** I've got this. | **2** Nice and cosy. | **3** Bed time it is. | **4** I am getting all my Zzz's tonight. | **5** Dear Bed, I love you. |
| **6** Tomorrow is another day. | **7** Do not disturb | **8** All I need is sleep. | **9** I am going to dream big tonight. | **10** INHALE EXHALE |
| **11** Keep calm and go to bed. | **12** I deserve more sleep. | **13** I will take over the world. Tomorrow. | **14** Charging time | **15** Sleep solves everything. |
| **16** My sleep game is strong. | **17** Status: In bed. | **18** I will feel so much better in the morning. | **19** ..but first sleep. | **20** 3...2...1 |
| **21** I can and I will. SLEEP. | **22** This one is for me. | **23** In bed on time? Check. | **24** The lion sleeps (well) tonight... | **25** Aaand pause. |
| **26** It's time. | **27** It will all be better tomorrow. | **28** Stronger in the morning. | **29** It makes a difference. | **30** Achievement Unlocked! |

## 48 Gladiator

Gladiators were the rockstars of the Roman world. They were the epitome of physical fitness, combat readiness and mental attitude. Training them was a full-time job that happened every single day. Gladiator is a challenge that asks you to develop and maintain the attitude and perseverance of a Gladiator. You won't find yourself in an arena, ready to battle to the death, but you will find yourself becoming more focused, disciplined and fitter.

# GLADIATOR

## 30-day challenge
© darebee.com

| | | | | |
|---|---|---|---|---|
| **1**<br>**40** punches<br>3 sets in total<br>20sec rest | **2**<br>**40 seconds**<br>one-arm plank<br>in one go | **3**<br>**10** lunges<br>3 sets in total<br>20sec rest | **4**<br>**40** punches<br>4 sets in total<br>20sec rest | **5**<br>**40 seconds**<br>one-arm plank<br>in one go |
| **6**<br>**10** lunges<br>4 sets in total<br>20sec rest | **7**<br>**60** punches<br>3 sets in total<br>20sec rest | **8**<br>**1 minute**<br>one-arm plank<br>in one go | **9**<br>**14** lunges<br>3 sets in total<br>20sec rest | **10**<br>**60** punches<br>4 sets in total<br>20sec rest |
| **11**<br>**1 minute**<br>one-arm plank<br>in one go | **12**<br>**14** lunges<br>4 sets in total<br>20sec rest | **13**<br>**80** punches<br>3 sets in total<br>20sec rest | **14**<br>**1min 20sec**<br>one-arm plank<br>in one go | **15**<br>**18** lunges<br>3 sets in total<br>20sec rest |
| **16**<br>**80** punches<br>4 sets in total<br>20sec rest | **17**<br>**1min 20sec**<br>one-arm plank<br>in one go | **18**<br>**18** lunges<br>4 sets in total<br>20sec rest | **19**<br>**100** punches<br>3 sets in total<br>20sec rest | **20**<br>**1min 40sec**<br>one-arm plank<br>in one go |
| **21**<br>**20** lunges<br>3 sets in total<br>20sec rest | **22**<br>**100** punches<br>4 sets in total<br>20sec rest | **23**<br>**1min 40sec**<br>one-arm plank<br>in one go | **24**<br>**20** lunges<br>4 sets in total<br>20sec rest | **25**<br>**120** punches<br>3 sets in total<br>20sec rest |
| **26**<br>**2 minutes**<br>one-arm plank<br>in one go | **27**<br>**22** lunges<br>3 sets in total<br>20sec rest | **28**<br>**120** punches<br>4 sets in total<br>20sec rest | **29**<br>**2 minutes**<br>one-arm plank<br>in one go | **30**<br>**22** lunges<br>4 sets in total<br>20sec rest |

# 49 Good Morning

How you start the day determines how you feel about yourself. How you feel about yourself affects the way you think, and then relate to the world. This is why it's important to start the day with a win. The Good Morning World! challenge helps you start each day with an instant win that will jumpstart your body and invigorate your mind. There will be a spring in your step. More than that, the small amount of impact you start the day with has been scientifically proven to boost circulation in the brain and body and help improve both cognitive and cardiovascular health. This halts cognitive decline as we age and helps prevent heart attacks.

Note: You can replace jumping jacks with step jacks.

# good morning, world!

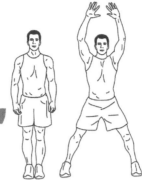

## 30-day challenge

Do jumping jacks
for 60 seconds non-stop
every morning, for 30 days

ⓒ darebee.com

| | | | | |
|---|---|---|---|---|
| **1** **60** seconds jumping jacks | **2** **60** seconds jumping jacks | **3** **60** seconds jumping jacks | **4** **60** seconds jumping jacks | **5** **60** seconds jumping jacks |
| **6** **60** seconds jumping jacks | **7** **60** seconds jumping jacks | **8** **60** seconds jumping jacks | **9** **60** seconds jumping jacks | **60** **60** seconds jumping jacks |
| **11** **60** seconds jumping jacks | **12** **60** seconds jumping jacks | **13** **60** seconds jumping jacks | **14** **60** seconds jumping jacks | **15** **60** seconds jumping jacks |
| **16** **60** seconds jumping jacks | **17** **60** seconds jumping jacks | **18** **60** seconds jumping jacks | **19** **60** seconds jumping jacks | **20** **60** seconds jumping jacks |
| **21** **60** seconds jumping jacks | **22** **60** seconds jumping jacks | **23** **60** seconds jumping jacks | **24** **60** seconds jumping jacks | **25** **60** seconds jumping jacks |
| **26** **60** seconds jumping jacks | **27** **60** seconds jumping jacks | **28** **60** seconds jumping jacks | **29** **60** seconds jumping jacks | **30** **60** seconds jumping jacks |

## 50 Hollow Hold

Isometric exercises, also known as static strength training, are contractions of a particular muscle for an extended period of time. The hollow hold works the body's anterior kinetic chain, the muscles in the front of the body; including abs, diaphragm, hip flexors, and quads. In addition to building strength, stability, and body control, it boasts back-friendly positioning by placing the body into a posterior pelvic tilt. The Hollow Hold challenge will make more than just your abs stronger. It will transform a major part of your body's functional strength.

# hollow hold

## 30-day challenge

© darebee.com

| | | | | |
|---|---|---|---|---|
| **1**<br>**20 seconds**<br>hollow hold | **2**<br>**20 seconds**<br>superman hold | **3**<br>**25 seconds**<br>hollow hold | **4**<br>**25 seconds**<br>superman hold | **5**<br>**30 seconds**<br>hollow hold |
| **6**<br>**30 seconds**<br>superman hold | **7**<br>**35 seconds**<br>hollow hold | **8**<br>**35 seconds**<br>superman hold | **9**<br>**40 seconds**<br>hollow hold | **10**<br>**40 seconds**<br>superman hold |
| **11**<br>**45 seconds**<br>hollow hold | **12**<br>**45 seconds**<br>superman hold | **13**<br>**50 seconds**<br>hollow hold | **14**<br>**50 seconds**<br>superman hold | **15**<br>**55 seconds**<br>hollow hold |
| **16**<br>**55 seconds**<br>superman hold | **17**<br>**60 seconds**<br>hollow hold | **18**<br>**60 seconds**<br>superman hold | **19**<br>**1min 10sec**<br>hollow hold | **20**<br>**1min 10sec**<br>superman hold |
| **21**<br>**1min 20sec**<br>hollow hold | **22**<br>**1min 20sec**<br>superman hold | **23**<br>**1min 30sec**<br>hollow hold | **24**<br>**1min 30sec**<br>superman hold | **25**<br>**1min 40sec**<br>hollow hold |
| **26**<br>**1min 40sec**<br>superman hold | **27**<br>**1min 50sec**<br>hollow hold | **28**<br>**1min 50sec**<br>superman hold | **29**<br>**2 minutes**<br>hollow hold | **30**<br>**2 minutes**<br>superman hold |

# 51 Home Marathon

The average time of a marathoner is 4:22:07 (9:59 minutes per mile pace) for men and 4:47:40 (10:58 minutes per mile pace) for women. A ten-minute run per day, over 30 days would see you complete 42.2 km hands down. High Knees are the biomechanical equivalent of sprinting. Sprinting requires high trajectory for the knees in order to generate the maximum amount of power over the shortest possible time and deliver speed in a given distance. Ten minutes of High Knees, performed in a form-perfect, virtually tireless manner delivers approximately 1,000 repetitions which, for our example, we shall assume are steps.

An average person walking at a fairly easy pace of 120 steps per minute takes 7,200 steps in an hour and covers 4.8km of distance. A marathon then (42.2km) is 63,300 steps or 2,110 steps per day over 30 days. Distance running however has a flatter trajectory than High Knees which leads us to a rough equivalent of 1 High Knee = 2.8 steps. You need to do just 750 form-perfect High Knees per day to cover the 42.2km of a marathon over a 30 day period.

The At-Home Marathon Challenge helps you perform this in a totally achievable way that will transform the biomechanical efficiency of your body, help you increase coordination, core strength, speed and power and endurance in just ten minutes a day.

Instructions: Set a timer and run for 10 minutes, every day for 30 days to complete a marathon run! For Extra Credit run all 10 minutes non-stop, without rest or breaks.

# at home MARATHON

## 30-day challenge

© darebee.com

| | | | | |
|---|---|---|---|---|
| **1** **10** minutes high knees | **2** **10** minutes high knees | **3** **10** minutes high knees | **4** **10** minutes high knees | **5** **10** minutes high knees |
| **6** **10** minutes high knees | **7** **10** minutes high knees | **8** **10** minutes high knees | **9** **10** minutes high knees | **10** **10** minutes high knees |
| **11** **10** minutes high knees | **12** **10** minutes high knees | **13** **10** minutes high knees | **14** **10** minutes high knees | **15** **10** minutes high knees |
| **16** **10** minutes high knees | **17** **10** minutes high knees | **18** **10** minutes high knees | **19** **10** minutes high knees | **20** **10** minutes high knees |
| **21** **10** minutes high knees | **22** **10** minutes high knees | **23** **10** minutes high knees | **24** **10** minutes high knees | **25** **10** minutes high knees |
| **26** **10** minutes high knees | **27** **10** minutes high knees | **28** **10** minutes high knees | **29** **10** minutes high knees | **30** **10** minutes high knees |

## 52 Homerun

High impact exercises strengthen the bones, help improve fascial fitness which, in turn improves resistance to fatigue from exercise and are key to developing strong, resilient muscles.

Homerun uses the body's own mass to help it become fitter and easier to manage. Over a month you will find yourself being lighter on your feet and more confident of your physical ability than before.

# home**run**

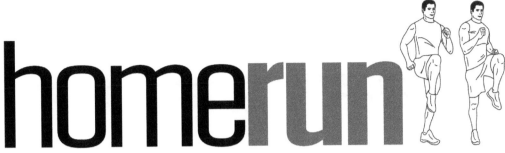

**30-DAY CHALLENGE**

up to 20 seconds rest between sets
each leg = 1 rep

© **darebee.com**

| | | | | |
|---|---|---|---|---|
| **1**<br>60 high knees<br>10 high knees<br>10 high knees | **2**<br>60 high knees<br>20 high knees<br>20 high knees | **3**<br>60 high knees<br>30 high knees<br>30 high knees | **4**<br>20 high knees<br>10 high knees<br>10 high knees | **5**<br>80 high knees<br>10 high knees<br>10 high knees |
| **6**<br>80 high knees<br>20 high knees<br>20 high knees | **7**<br>80 high knees<br>30 high knees<br>30 high knees | **8**<br>20 high knees<br>10 high knees<br>10 high knees | **9**<br>100 high knees<br>10 high knees<br>10 high knees | **10**<br>100 high knees<br>20 high knees<br>20 high knees |
| **11**<br>100 high knees<br>30 high knees<br>30 high knees | **12**<br>20 high knees<br>10 high knees<br>10 high knees | **13**<br>120 high knees<br>10 high knees<br>10 high knees | **14**<br>120 high knees<br>20 high knees<br>20 high knees | **15**<br>120 high knees<br>30 high knees<br>30 high knees |
| **16**<br>20 high knees<br>10 high knees<br>10 high knees | **17**<br>140 high knees<br>10 high knees<br>10 high knees | **18**<br>140 high knees<br>20 high knees<br>20 high knees | **19**<br>140 high knees<br>30 high knees<br>30 high knees | **20**<br>20 high knees<br>10 high knees<br>10 high knees |
| **21**<br>160 high knees<br>10 high knees<br>10 high knees | **22**<br>160 high knees<br>20 high knees<br>20 high knees | **23**<br>160 high knees<br>30 high knees<br>30 high knees | **24**<br>20 high knees<br>10 high knees<br>10 high knees | **25**<br>180 high knees<br>10 high knees<br>10 high knees |
| **26**<br>180 high knees<br>20 high knees<br>20 high knees | **27**<br>180 high knees<br>30 high knees<br>30 high knees | **28**<br>20 high knees<br>10 high knees<br>10 high knees | **29**<br>200 high knees<br>10 high knees<br>10 high knees | **30**<br>200 high knees<br>20 high knees<br>20 high knees |

## 53 Impact

High-impact workouts are really challenging. They force the body to improve fascial fitness so the connective tissue between organs becomes denser and more absorbent of vibrations. In turn this helps the muscles become more durable as they get factigued less.

More than that, high-impact exercises improve the vertical force the body can apply improving its ability to jump higher and land easier.

# IMPACT

## 30-DAY CHALLENGE

split total reps into manageable sets

© darebee.com

| | | | | |
|---|---|---|---|---|
| **1**<br>20 jump squats<br>20 plank jump-ins<br>20 basic burpees | **2**<br>**20**<br>calf raises | **3**<br>**20**<br>jump knee-tucks | **4**<br>60 seconds<br>plank hold | **5**<br>40 jump squats<br>40 plank jump-ins<br>40 basic burpees |
| **6**<br>**40**<br>calf raises | **7**<br>**40**<br>jump knee-tucks | **8**<br>2 minutes<br>plank hold | **9**<br>50 jump squats<br>50 plank jump-ins<br>50 basic burpees | **10**<br>**50**<br>calf raises |
| **11**<br>**50**<br>jump knee-tucks | **12**<br>4 minutes<br>plank hold | **13**<br>60 jump squats<br>60 plank jump-ins<br>60 basic burpees | **14**<br>**60**<br>calf raises | **15**<br>**60**<br>jump knee-tucks |
| **16**<br>6 minutes<br>plank hold | **17**<br>70 jump squats<br>70 plank jump-ins<br>70 basic burpees | **18**<br>**70**<br>calf raises | **19**<br>**70**<br>jump knee-tucks | **20**<br>8 minutes<br>plank hold |
| **21**<br>80 jump squats<br>80 plank jump-ins<br>80 basic burpees | **22**<br>**80**<br>calf raises | **23**<br>**80**<br>jump knee-tucks | **24**<br>10 minutes<br>plank hold | **25**<br>100 jump squats<br>100 plank jump-ins<br>100 basic burpees |
| **26**<br>**100**<br>calf raises | **27**<br>**100**<br>jump knee-tucks | **28**<br>12 minutes<br>plank hold | **29**<br>120 jump squats<br>120 plank jump-ins<br>120 basic burpees | **30**<br>**120**<br>calf raises |

## 54 Impossible Abs

Three distinct exercises, three sets a day and thirty days. The Impossible Abs challenge will transform the way you sit, stand, walk, run and jump by strengthening each of the four different muscle groups that make up the abs set. As a result you will feel different not just about the way you move and the way you look but also the way you approach physical activity of every type. Use this to level up if you've been experiencing a plateau in your fitness journey or use it as one more means through which you get closer and closer to the physically better version of you.

Note: All reps are given in total so 10 side bridges = 5 per side.

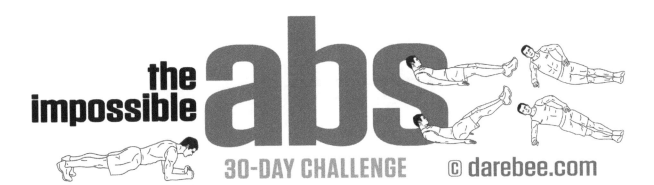

# the impossible abs

## 30-DAY CHALLENGE  © darebee.com

| 1 | 2 | 3 | 4 | 5 |
|---|---|---|---|---|
| **8 leg raises**<br>**8 side bridges**<br>3 sets \| 30sec rest | **20 seconds**<br>elbow plank hold<br>3 sets \| 30sec rest | **8 leg raises**<br>**8 side bridges**<br>3 sets \| 30sec rest | **20 seconds**<br>elbow plank hold<br>3 sets \| 30sec rest | **10 leg raises**<br>**10 side bridges**<br>3 sets \| 30sec rest |

| 6 | 7 | 8 | 9 | 10 |
|---|---|---|---|---|
| **25 seconds**<br>elbow plank hold<br>3 sets \| 30sec rest | **10 leg raises**<br>**10 side bridges**<br>3 sets \| 30sec rest | **25 seconds**<br>elbow plank hold<br>3 sets \| 30sec rest | **12 leg raises**<br>**12 side bridges**<br>3 sets \| 30sec rest | **30 seconds**<br>elbow plank hold<br>3 sets \| 30sec rest |

| 11 | 12 | 13 | 14 | 15 |
|---|---|---|---|---|
| **12 leg raises**<br>**12 side bridges**<br>3 sets \| 30sec rest | **30 seconds**<br>elbow plank hold<br>3 sets \| 30sec rest | **14 leg raises**<br>**14 side bridges**<br>3 sets \| 30sec rest | **35 seconds**<br>elbow plank hold<br>3 sets \| 30sec rest | **14 leg raises**<br>**14 side bridges**<br>3 sets \| 30sec rest |

| 16 | 17 | 18 | 19 | 20 |
|---|---|---|---|---|
| **35 seconds**<br>elbow plank hold<br>3 sets \| 30sec rest | **16 leg raises**<br>**16 side bridges**<br>3 sets \| 30sec rest | **40 seconds**<br>elbow plank hold<br>3 sets \| 30sec rest | **16 leg raises**<br>**16 side bridges**<br>3 sets \| 30sec rest | **40 seconds**<br>elbow plank hold<br>3 sets \| 30sec rest |

| 21 | 22 | 23 | 24 | 25 |
|---|---|---|---|---|
| **18 leg raises**<br>**18 side bridges**<br>3 sets \| 30sec rest | **45 seconds**<br>elbow plank hold<br>3 sets \| 30sec rest | **18 leg raises**<br>**18 side bridges**<br>3 sets \| 30sec rest | **45 seconds**<br>elbow plank hold<br>3 sets \| 30sec rest | **20 leg raises**<br>**20 side bridges**<br>3 sets \| 30sec rest |

| 26 | 27 | 28 | 29 | 30 |
|---|---|---|---|---|
| **50 seconds**<br>elbow plank hold<br>3 sets \| 30sec rest | **20 leg raises**<br>**20 side bridges**<br>3 sets \| 30sec rest | **50 seconds**<br>elbow plank hold<br>3 sets \| 30sec rest | **22 leg raises**<br>**22 side bridges**<br>3 sets \| 30sec rest | **60 seconds**<br>elbow plank hold<br>3 sets \| 30sec rest |

## 55 Iron Core

A strong core helps you sit, stand, run, jump and kick better. It can make you resistant to fatigue, nimble on your feet and more powerful in your athleticism. the Iron Core challenge helps you develop a strong core. A strong core will help you do everything else differently; even your posture will change. Then everything will change for you. And it all starts so easily.

# IRON CORE

## 30-DAY CHALLENGE

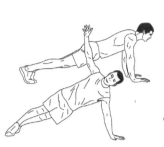
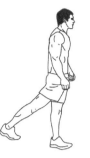
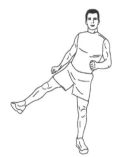

© darebee.com

| | | | | |
|---|---|---|---|---|
| **1**<br>**10 plank rotations**<br>3 sets<br>30 seconds rest | **2**<br>**20 seconds**<br>leg raise hold<br>side leg raise hold | **3**<br>**10 plank rotations**<br>3 sets<br>30 seconds rest | **4**<br>**20 seconds**<br>leg raise hold<br>side leg raise hold | **5**<br>**12 plank rotations**<br>3 sets<br>30 seconds rest |
| **6**<br>**30 seconds**<br>leg raise hold<br>side leg raise hold | **7**<br>**12 plank rotations**<br>3 sets<br>30 seconds rest | **8**<br>**30 seconds**<br>leg raise hold<br>side leg raise hold | **9**<br>**14 plank rotations**<br>3 sets<br>30 seconds rest | **10**<br>**40 seconds**<br>leg raise hold<br>side leg raise hold |
| **11**<br>**14 plank rotations**<br>3 sets<br>30 seconds rest | **12**<br>**40 seconds**<br>leg raise hold<br>side leg raise hold | **13**<br>**16 plank rotations**<br>3 sets<br>30 seconds rest | **14**<br>**50 seconds**<br>leg raise hold<br>side leg raise hold | **15**<br>**16 plank rotations**<br>3 sets<br>30 seconds rest |
| **16**<br>**50 seconds**<br>leg raise hold<br>side leg raise hold | **17**<br>**18 plank rotations**<br>3 sets<br>30 seconds rest | **18**<br>**60 seconds**<br>leg raise hold<br>side leg raise hold | **19**<br>**18 plank rotations**<br>3 sets<br>30 seconds rest | **20**<br>**60 seconds**<br>leg raise hold<br>side leg raise hold |
| **21**<br>**20 plank rotations**<br>3 sets<br>30 seconds rest | **22**<br>**1min 10sec**<br>leg raise hold<br>side leg raise hold | **23**<br>**20 plank rotations**<br>3 sets<br>30 seconds rest | **24**<br>**1min 10sec**<br>leg raise hold<br>side leg raise hold | **25**<br>**22 plank rotations**<br>3 sets<br>30 seconds rest |
| **26**<br>**1min 20sec**<br>leg raise hold<br>side leg raise hold | **27**<br>**22 plank rotations**<br>3 sets<br>30 seconds rest | **28**<br>**1min 20sec**<br>leg raise hold<br>side leg raise hold | **29**<br>**24 plank rotations**<br>3 sets<br>30 seconds rest | **30**<br>**1min 30sec**<br>leg raise hold<br>side leg raise hold |

## 56 Iron Glutes

The glutes are stabilizers. Their primary role is to stabilize the plevis and the hip so the body can function freely. The functions of the three different muscle groups that form the glutes include extension, abduction, external rotation, and internal rotation of the hip joint.

Glutes are frequently referred to as the strongest muscle in the body. They help us stay erect and play a pivotal role in generating physical power when we run, jump, kick and punch.

# IRON GLUTES

## 30-DAY CHALLENGE

© darebee.com

| | | | | |
|---|---|---|---|---|
| **1**<br>20 side kicks<br>1min rest<br>2 sets | **2**<br>8 shrimp squats<br>1min rest<br>2 sets | **3**<br>**80**<br>side kicks<br>throughout the day | **4**<br>10 shrimp squats<br>1min rest<br>2 sets | **5**<br>24 side kicks<br>1min rest<br>2 sets |
| **6**<br>12 shrimp squats<br>1min rest<br>2 sets | **7**<br>**100**<br>side kicks<br>throughout the day | **8**<br>8 shrimp squats<br>1min rest<br>3 sets | **9**<br>20 side kicks<br>1min rest<br>3 sets | **10**<br>10 shrimp squats<br>1min rest<br>3 sets |
| **11**<br>**120**<br>side kicks<br>throughout the day | **12**<br>12 shrimp squats<br>1min rest<br>3 sets | **13**<br>24 side kicks<br>1min rest<br>3 sets | **14**<br>8 shrimp squats<br>1min rest<br>4 sets | **15**<br>**140**<br>side kicks<br>throughout the day |
| **16**<br>10 shrimp squats<br>1min rest<br>4 sets | **17**<br>20 side kicks<br>1min rest<br>4 sets | **18**<br>12 shrimp squats<br>1min rest<br>4 sets | **19**<br>**160**<br>side kicks<br>throughout the day | **20**<br>8 shrimp squats<br>1min rest<br>5 sets |
| **21**<br>24 side kicks<br>1min rest<br>4 sets | **22**<br>10 shrimp squats<br>1min rest<br>5 sets | **23**<br>**180**<br>side kicks<br>throughout the day | **24**<br>12 shrimp squats<br>1min rest<br>5 sets | **25**<br>20 side kicks<br>1min rest<br>5 sets |
| **26**<br>8 shrimp squats<br>1min rest<br>6 sets | **27**<br>**200**<br>side kicks<br>throughout the day | **28**<br>10 shrimp squats<br>1min rest<br>6 sets | **29**<br>24 side kicks<br>1min rest<br>5 sets | **30**<br>12 shrimp squats<br>1min rest<br>6 sets |

## 57    Iron Will

It takes courage to take that first step in the right direction but it takes an iron will to keep on going. Take up the challenge and see it through - forge your will as you forge your muscles.

Every other day is a maintenance and recovery day with only 30 lunges. All reps are given in total so 30 lunges = 15 per leg. The total number of reps is a total for the day.

# IRON WILL

## 30-day challenge

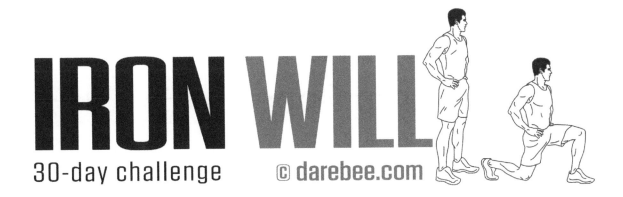

© darebee.com

| | | | | |
|---|---|---|---|---|
| **1** 30 lunges | **2** 60 lunges | **3** 30 lunges | **4** 70 lunges | **5** 30 lunges |
| **6** 80 lunges | **7** 30 lunges | **8** 90 lunges | **9** 30 lunges | **10** 100 lunges |
| **11** 30 lunges | **12** 110 lunges | **13** 30 lunges | **14** 120 lunges | **15** 30 lunges |
| **16** 130 lunges | **17** 30 lunges | **18** 140 lunges | **19** 30 lunges | **20** 150 lunges |
| **21** 30 lunges | **22** 160 lunges | **23** 30 lunges | **24** 170 lunges | **25** 30 lunges |
| **26** 180 lunges | **27** 30 lunges | **28** 190 lunges | **29** 30 lunges | **30** 200 lunges |

## 58 | Jump Rope

Jump Rope is a seemingly simple high-impact challenge. Yet it does incredible things. For a start it promotes active hand/eye coordination. It then encourages the growth of neurons in the brain as fresh connections are required to coordinate the motor neuron function that keeps the swinging of the jump rope in sync with hopping in order to avoid it.

Finally, it helps promote bone density, cardiovascular health and it can even increase aerobic endurance.

# JUMP ROPE

## 30-DAY CHALLENGE

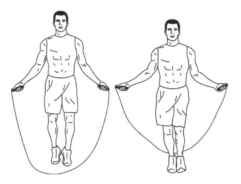

© darebee.com

| | | | | |
|---|---|---|---|---|
| **1**<br>1 min skips<br>1 min rest<br>3 sets in total | **2**<br>4 min in total<br>throughout<br>the day | **3**<br>2 min skips<br>non-stop | **4**<br>1 min skips<br>1 min rest<br>3 sets in total | **5**<br>**200 skips**<br>one workout |
| **6**<br>1 min skips<br>1 min rest<br>3 sets in total | **7**<br>4 min in total<br>throughout<br>the day | **8**<br>2 min skips<br>non-stop | **9**<br>1 min skips<br>1 min rest<br>3 sets in total | **10**<br>**400 skips**<br>one workout |
| **11**<br>1 min skips<br>1 min rest<br>4 sets in total | **12**<br>6 min in total<br>throughout<br>the day | **13**<br>3 min skips<br>non-stop | **14**<br>1 min skips<br>1 min rest<br>4 sets in total | **15**<br>**450 skips**<br>one workout |
| **16**<br>1 min skips<br>1 min rest<br>4 sets in total | **17**<br>6 min in total<br>throughout<br>the day | **18**<br>3 min skips<br>non-stop | **19**<br>1 min skips<br>1 min rest<br>4 sets in total | **20**<br>**600 skips**<br>one workout |
| **21**<br>1 min skips<br>1 min rest<br>4 sets in total | **22**<br>8 min in total<br>throughout<br>the day | **23**<br>4 min skips<br>non-stop | **24**<br>1 min skips<br>1 min rest<br>4 sets in total | **25**<br>**800 skips**<br>one workout |
| **26**<br>1 min skips<br>1 min rest<br>5 sets in total | **27**<br>10 min in total<br>throughout<br>the day | **28**<br>4 min skips<br>non-stop | **29**<br>1 min skips<br>1 min rest<br>5 sets in total | **30**<br>**1000 skips**<br>one workout |

## 59  Kicks & Punches

Kicks and punches challenge the body at many levels. They promote close coordination of the entire kinetic chain that transforms strength and speed into power. They help muscles become more flexible and coordinated, strengthen the core and improve agility, plus they activate both your cardiovascular and aerobic systems.

# KICKS & PUNCHES

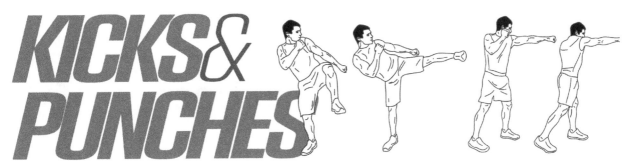

## 30-DAY CHALLENGE

© darebee.com

| | | | | |
|---|---|---|---|---|
| **1**<br>**20** side kicks<br>3 sets in total<br>30sec rest | **2**<br>**20** punches<br>3 sets in total<br>30sec rest | **3**<br>**100** side kicks<br>in total<br>throughout the day | **4**<br>**100** punches<br>in total<br>throughout the day | **5**<br>**20** side kicks<br>4 sets in total<br>30sec rest |
| **6**<br>**20** punches<br>4 sets in total<br>30sec rest | **7**<br>**150** side kicks<br>in total<br>throughout the day | **8**<br>**150** punches<br>in total<br>throughout the day | **9**<br>**30** side kicks<br>3 sets in total<br>30sec rest | **10**<br>**30** punches<br>3 sets in total<br>30sec rest |
| **11**<br>**200** side kicks<br>in total<br>throughout the day | **12**<br>**200** punches<br>in total<br>throughout the day | **13**<br>**30** side kicks<br>4 sets in total<br>30sec rest | **14**<br>**30** punches<br>4 sets in total<br>30sec rest | **15**<br>**250** side kicks<br>in total<br>throughout the day |
| **16**<br>**250** punches<br>in total<br>throughout the day | **17**<br>**40** side kicks<br>3 sets in total<br>30sec rest | **18**<br>**40** punches<br>3 sets in total<br>30sec rest | **19**<br>**300** side kicks<br>in total<br>throughout the day | **20**<br>**300** punches<br>in total<br>throughout the day |
| **21**<br>**40** side kicks<br>4 sets in total<br>30sec rest | **22**<br>**40** punches<br>4 sets in total<br>30sec rest | **23**<br>**350** side kicks<br>in total<br>throughout the day | **24**<br>**350** punches<br>in total<br>throughout the day | **25**<br>**50** side kicks<br>3 sets in total<br>30sec rest |
| **26**<br>**50** punches<br>3 sets in total<br>30sec rest | **27**<br>**400** side kicks<br>in total<br>throughout the day | **28**<br>**400** punches<br>in total<br>throughout the day | **29**<br>**50** side kicks<br>4 sets in total<br>30sec rest | **30**<br>**50** punches<br>4 sets in total<br>30sec rest |

## 60    Knee Push-Ups

Push-ups are the perfect exercise. They help develop strong arms and shoulders. They work out the chest and abs. They challenge the core; strengthen neck muscles, recruit the tendons of the hips and lower back and even work the quads and glutes. Yet not everyone can do them and you can't do them the question is, how do you even start? The Knee Push-Ups Challenge helps you get where you want to by allowing you to develop all the same muscle groups at a gradual pace with a lighter load. If you can't yet do outright push-ups and want to get to that exulted state then this is the Challenge to start with. It will change how you feel about yourself. More than that, it will change what you can physically do.

What it works: chest, tricep and shoulders.

The challenge is suitable for both men and women. It'll help you tighten up your chest muscles, shaping and lifting your pecs (breasts).

# knee push-ups

## 30-DAY CHALLENGE

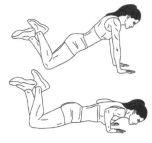

© darebee.com

| 1 | 2 | 3 | 4 | 5 |
|---|---|---|---|---|
| **5 knee push-ups** <br> 3 sets <br> 30 seconds rest | **20 seconds** <br> knee push-up <br> hold | **5 knee push-ups** <br> 3 sets <br> 30 seconds rest | **20 seconds** <br> knee push-up <br> hold | **6 knee push-ups** <br> 3 sets <br> 30 seconds rest |
| **6** | **7** | **8** | **9** | **10** |
| **25 seconds** <br> knee push-up <br> hold | **6 knee push-ups** <br> 3 sets <br> 30 seconds rest | **25 seconds** <br> knee push-up <br> hold | **7 knee push-ups** <br> 3 sets <br> 30 seconds rest | **30 seconds** <br> knee push-up <br> hold |
| **11** | **12** | **13** | **14** | **15** |
| **7 knee push-ups** <br> 3 sets <br> 30 seconds rest | **30 seconds** <br> knee push-up <br> hold | **8 knee push-ups** <br> 3 sets <br> 30 seconds rest | **35 seconds** <br> knee push-up <br> hold | **8 knee push-ups** <br> 3 sets <br> 30 seconds rest |
| **16** | **17** | **18** | **19** | **20** |
| **35 seconds** <br> knee push-up <br> hold | **9 knee push-ups** <br> 3 sets <br> 30 seconds rest | **40 seconds** <br> knee push-up <br> hold | **9 knee push-ups** <br> 3 sets <br> 30 seconds rest | **40 seconds** <br> knee push-up <br> hold |
| **21** | **22** | **23** | **24** | **25** |
| **10 knee push-ups** <br> 3 sets <br> 30 seconds rest | **45 seconds** <br> knee push-up <br> hold | **10 knee push-ups** <br> 3 sets <br> 30 seconds rest | **45 seconds** <br> knee push-up <br> hold | **11 knee push-ups** <br> 3 sets <br> 30 seconds rest |
| **26** | **27** | **28** | **29** | **30** |
| **50 seconds** <br> knee push-up <br> hold | **11 knee push-ups** <br> 3 sets <br> 30 seconds rest | **50 seconds** <br> knee push-up <br> hold | **12 knee push-ups** <br> 3 sets <br> 30 seconds rest | **60 seconds** <br> knee push-up <br> hold |

## 61 Legs Of Steel

Powerful quads translate the pull of the planet on the mass of your body into high-quality energy you can use for your own purpose. The legs of Steel challenge will help you level up by acquiring the kind of lower body strength that helps you stand, walk, run, jump and kick better. All you have to do is start one day one and come out transformed at the end of day thirty.

# legs of steel
## *of* steel
### 30-DAY CHALLENGE

© darebee.com

| 1 | 2 | 3 | 4 | 5 |
|---|---|---|---|---|
| **22** lunges<br>**20sec** rest<br>3 sets | **12** side lunges<br>**20sec** rest<br>3 sets | **22** lunges<br>**20sec** rest<br>3 sets | **12** side lunges<br>**20sec** rest<br>3 sets | **22** lunges<br>**20sec** rest<br>3 sets |
| 6 | 7 | 8 | 9 | 10 |
| **12** side lunges<br>**20sec** rest<br>3 sets | **24** lunges<br>**20sec** rest<br>3 sets | **14** side lunges<br>**20sec** rest<br>3 sets | **24** lunges<br>**20sec** rest<br>3 sets | **14** side lunges<br>**20sec** rest<br>3 sets |
| 11 | 12 | 13 | 14 | 15 |
| **24** lunges<br>**20sec** rest<br>3 sets | **14** side lunges<br>**20sec** rest<br>3 sets | **26** lunges<br>**20sec** rest<br>3 sets | **16** side lunges<br>**20sec** rest<br>3 sets | **26** lunges<br>**20sec** rest<br>3 sets |
| 16 | 17 | 18 | 19 | 20 |
| **16** side lunges<br>**20sec** rest<br>3 sets | **26** lunges<br>**20sec** rest<br>3 sets | **16** side lunges<br>**20sec** rest<br>3 sets | **28** lunges<br>**20sec** rest<br>3 sets | **18** side lunges<br>**20sec** rest<br>3 sets |
| 21 | 22 | 23 | 24 | 25 |
| **28** lunges<br>**20sec** rest<br>3 sets | **18** side lunges<br>**20sec** rest<br>3 sets | **28** lunges<br>**20sec** rest<br>3 sets | **18** side lunges<br>**20sec** rest<br>3 sets | **30** lunges<br>**20sec** rest<br>3 sets |
| 26 | 27 | 28 | 28 | 30 |
| **20** side lunges<br>**20sec** rest<br>3 sets | **30** lunges<br>**20sec** rest<br>3 sets | **20** side lunges<br>**20sec** rest<br>3 sets | **30** lunges<br>**20sec** rest<br>3 sets | **20** side lunges<br>**20sec** rest<br>3 sets |

## 62    Makeover

What if you had the chance for a physical makeover that would amp-up your ability to run fast, tire less and maintain near-perfect form? Makeover uses seemingly simple exercises to help you attain greater control over your body, greater arm/leg coordination and stronger tendons. Over thirty days you will feel the difference targeted exercises make to your overall athletic ability.

# make over

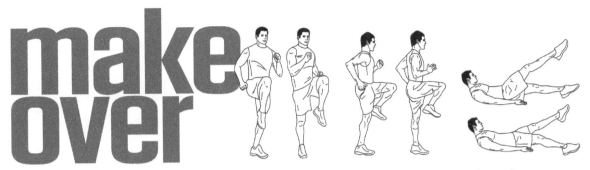

**30-DAY CHALLENGE**     **burn body fat, build abs**     © darebee.com

| | | | | |
|---|---|---|---|---|
| **1**<br>30sec high knees<br>30sec march steps<br>3 sets | no rest | **2**<br>**10**<br>flutter kicks<br>3 sets | 2min rest | **3**<br>30sec high knees<br>30sec march steps<br>4 sets | no rest | **4**<br>**10**<br>flutter kicks<br>4 sets | 2min rest | **5**<br>30sec high knees<br>30sec march steps<br>5 sets | no rest |
| **6**<br>**10**<br>flutter kicks<br>5 sets | 2min rest | **7**<br>30sec high knees<br>30sec march steps<br>6 sets | no rest | **8**<br>**20**<br>flutter kicks<br>3 sets | 2min rest | **9**<br>30sec high knees<br>30sec march steps<br>7 sets | no rest | **10**<br>**20**<br>flutter kicks<br>4 sets | 2min rest |
| **11**<br>30sec high knees<br>30sec march steps<br>8 sets | no rest | **12**<br>**20**<br>flutter kicks<br>5 sets | 2min rest | **13**<br>30sec high knees<br>30sec march steps<br>9 sets | no rest | **14**<br>**30**<br>flutter kicks<br>3 sets | 2min rest | **15**<br>30sec high knees<br>30sec march steps<br>10 sets | no rest |
| **16**<br>**30**<br>flutter kicks<br>4 sets | 2min rest | **17**<br>1min high knees<br>1min march steps<br>5 sets | no rest | **18**<br>**30**<br>flutter kicks<br>5 sets | 2min rest | **19**<br>1min high knees<br>1min march steps<br>6 sets | no rest | **20**<br>**40**<br>flutter kicks<br>3 sets | 2min rest |
| **21**<br>1min high knees<br>1min march steps<br>7 sets | no rest | **22**<br>**40**<br>flutter kicks<br>4 sets | 2min rest | **23**<br>1min high knees<br>1min march steps<br>8 sets | no rest | **24**<br>**40**<br>flutter kicks<br>5 sets | 2min rest | **25**<br>1min high knees<br>1min march steps<br>9 sets | no rest |
| **26**<br>**50**<br>flutter kicks<br>3 sets | 2min rest | **27**<br>1min high knees<br>1min march steps<br>10 sets | no rest | **28**<br>**50**<br>flutter kicks<br>4 sets | 2min rest | **29**<br>2min high knees<br>1min march steps<br>7 sets | no rest | **30**<br>**50**<br>flutter kicks<br>5 sets | 2min rest |

# 63  Meditation

Neuroscientific research has shown that meditation literally rewires the brain and allows you to change the perspective of your inner world. This creates a stronger sense of inner peace, a clearer sense of purpose and a mental clarity that allows you to face every potential crisis in a measured, concerted way.

## Backup & Restore

DAREBEE WORKOUT
© darebee.com

slowly move from one position to the next; hold each pose for 4 seconds

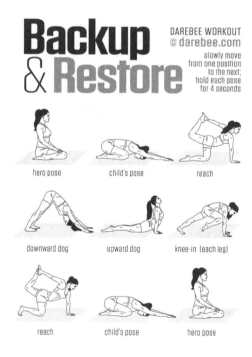

hero pose    child's pose    reach

downward dog    upward dog    knee-in (each leg)

reach    child's pose    hero pose

## OM Mantra

Imagine the sound of OM Mantra internally, in the mind only, making no external sound. Allow the mantra to flow with the breath:

Exhale "OMmmmmmmm..."
Inhale "OMmmmmmmm..."

Exhale "OMmmmmmmm..."
Inhale "OMmmmmmmm..."

Exhale "OMmmmmmmm..."
Inhale "OMmmmmmmm..."

# meditation

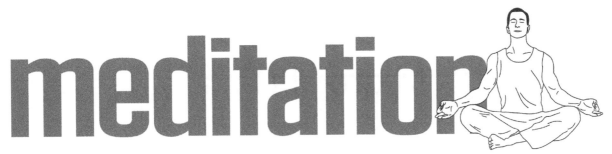

**30-DAY CHALLENGE**

© darebee.com

| | | | | |
|---|---|---|---|---|
| **1**<br>5 minutes | **2**<br>1-minute Equal Breathing +<br>5 minutes | **3**<br>Backup & Restore Workout +<br>5 minutes | **4**<br>5 minutes<br>+ OM mantra | **5**<br>5 minutes |
| **6**<br>1-minute Equal Breathing +<br>5 minutes | **7**<br>Backup & Restore Workout +<br>5 minutes | **8**<br>5 minutes | **9**<br>5 minutes<br>+ OM mantra | **10**<br>1-minute Equal Breathing +<br>5 minutes |
| **11**<br>Backup & Restore Workout +<br>10 minutes | **12**<br>10 minutes | **13**<br>10 minutes<br>+ OM mantra | **14**<br>1-minute Equal Breathing +<br>10 minutes | **15**<br>Backup & Restore Workout +<br>10 minutes |
| **16**<br>10 minutes | **17**<br>10 minutes<br>+ OM mantra | **18**<br>1-minute Equal Breathing +<br>10 minutes | **19**<br>Backup & Restore Workout +<br>10 minutes | **20**<br>10 minutes |
| **21**<br>15 minutes<br>+ OM mantra | **22**<br>1-minute Equal Breathing +<br>15 minutes | **23**<br>Backup & Restore Workout +<br>15 minutes | **24**<br>15 minutes | **25**<br>15 minutes<br>+ OM mantra |
| **26**<br>1-minute Equal Breathing +<br>15 minutes | **27**<br>Backup & Restore Workout +<br>15 minutes | **28**<br>15 minutes | **29**<br>15 minutes<br>+ OM mantra | **30**<br>20 minutes |

## 64    Micro HIIT

The science behind the effectiveness of micro-workouts shows that done consistency, over time, they trigger the body's adaptive response helping muscles get stronger and fitness base levels to be recalibrated. Micro HIIT is a challenge that helps you get further in your fitness journey with less effort.

# micro HIIT

## 30-DAY CHALLENGE

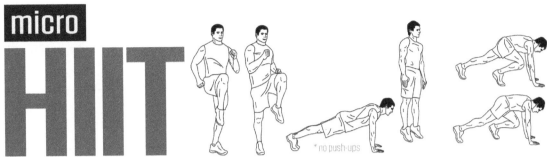

*no push-ups

© darebee.com

**1**
10sec high knees
10sec climbers
10sec high knees
60sec rest | 3 sets

**2**
10sec burpees
10sec rest
10sec burpees
60sec rest | 3 sets

**3**
10sec slow climbers
10sec fast climbers
60sec rest | 3 sets

**4**
20sec burpees
20sec rest | 3 sets

**5**
10sec high knees
10sec climbers
10sec high knees
60sec rest | 4 sets

**6**
10sec burpees
10sec rest
10sec burpees
60sec rest | 4 sets

**7**
10sec slow climbers
10sec fast climbers
60sec rest | 4 sets

**8**
20sec burpees
20sec rest | 3 sets

**9**
20sec high knees
20sec climbers
20sec high knees
60sec rest | 3 sets

**10**
20sec burpees
20sec rest
20sec burpees
60sec rest | 3 sets

**11**
20sec slow climbers
20sec fast climbers
60sec rest | 3 sets

**12**
20sec burpees
20sec rest | 4 sets

**13**
20sec high knees
20sec climbers
20sec high knees
60sec rest | 4 sets

**14**
20sec burpees
20sec rest
20sec burpees
60sec rest | 4 sets

**15**
20sec slow climbers
20sec fast climbers
60sec rest | 4 sets

**16**
20sec burpees
20sec rest | 4 sets

**17**
20sec high knees
20sec climbers
20sec high knees
60sec rest | 5 sets

**18**
20sec burpees
20sec rest
20sec burpees
60sec rest | 5 sets

**19**
20sec slow climbers
20sec fast climbers
60sec rest | 5 sets

**20**
20sec burpees
20sec rest | 5 sets

**21**
20sec high knees
20sec climbers
20sec high knees
40sec rest | 5 sets

**22**
20sec burpees
20sec rest
20sec burpees
40sec rest | 4 sets

**23**
20sec slow climbers
20sec fast climbers
40sec rest | 5 sets

**24**
20sec burpees
20sec rest | 5 sets

**25**
20sec high knees
20sec climbers
20sec high knees
40sec rest | 6 sets

**26**
20sec burpees
20sec rest
20sec burpees
40sec rest | 5 sets

**27**
20sec slow climbers
20sec fast climbers
20sec rest | 5 sets

**28**
20sec burpees
20sec rest | 6 sets

**29**
20sec high knees
20sec climbers
20sec high knees
20sec rest | 6 sets

**30**
20sec burpees
20sec rest
20sec burpees
20sec rest | 5 sets

## 65 Multiplank

Planks strengthen the core, shoulders, lower back, glutes, quads and chest and shoulders. All, in two-minute lots. The multi-plank challenge helps you develop strong abs and core, plus over a month you get to also develop the kind of mental discipline that transforms you from the inside out.

Hold each plank for 2 minutes in total (1 minute per side).

# 2-minute multiplank

**30-DAY CHALLENGE**

© darebee.com

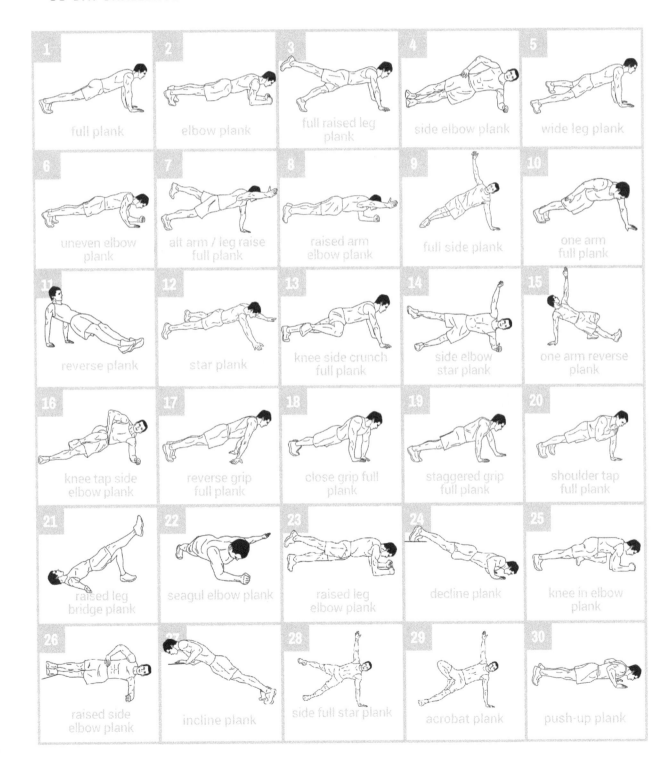

| | | | | |
|---|---|---|---|---|
| **1** full plank | **2** elbow plank | **3** full raised leg plank | **4** side elbow plank | **5** wide leg plank |
| **6** uneven elbow plank | **7** alt arm / leg raise full plank | **8** raised arm elbow plank | **9** full side plank | **10** one arm full plank |
| **11** reverse plank | **12** star plank | **13** knee side crunch full plank | **14** side elbow star plank | **15** one arm reverse plank |
| **16** knee tap side elbow plank | **17** reverse grip full plank | **18** close grip full plank | **19** staggered grip full plank | **20** shoulder tap full plank |
| **21** raised leg bridge plank | **22** seagul elbow plank | **23** raised leg elbow plank | **24** decline plank | **25** knee in elbow plank |
| **26** raised side elbow plank | **27** incline plank | **28** side full star plank | **29** acrobat plank | **30** push-up plank |

# 66 Negative Pull-Up

In the negative pull-ups challenge you get to challenge gravity itself. Muscles grow stronger when contracting eccentrically (they lengthen) instead of when contracting concentrically (they shorten, what we call the usual "flexing of muscles"). Negative pull-ups require you to start from a full pull up position and slowly go backwards until you find yourself hanging, arms fully extended or what we call the dead hang position. The eccentric motion of the muscles (i.e. the lengthening of muscle fibers) generates more force at a lower metabolic rate (probably due to titin engagement in muscle lengthening). In addition, it engages, a lot of additional muscles such as core, abs, upper back and even lower back as the body's downward motion needs to be stabilized and controlled. The force exerted by the muscles recruits tendons in an active stretching capacity lengthening them as the muscles stretch and increasing their own strength and stability.

The dead hang position has additional strength benefits. In the first instance it increases grip strength which has become an important predictor of overall health and strength. It also helps develop fascial fitness which has important implications in the body's ability to tire from exercise and to translate muscle strength into power and explosive movement. At the end of the 30-day Negative Pull-Ups challenge you will feel in yourself a variety of changes in strength and endurance.

# negative pull-ups

## 30-DAY CHALLENGE

© darebee.com

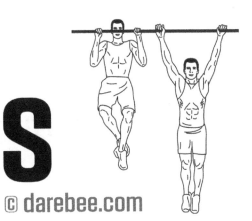

| | | | | |
|---|---|---|---|---|
| **1**<br>2 negative pull-up<br>1 negative pull-up<br>1 negative pull-up<br>up to 2min rest | **2**<br>**10sec** dead hang<br>2 sets in total<br>up to 2min rest | **3**<br>2 negative pull-ups<br>2 negative pull-up<br>1 negative pull-up<br>up to 2min rest | **4**<br>**10sec** dead hang<br>2 sets in total<br>up to 2min rest | **5**<br>2 negative pull-ups<br>2 negative pull-ups<br>2 negative pull-up<br>up to 2min rest |
| **6**<br>**10sec** dead hang<br>3 sets in total<br>up to 2min rest | **7**<br>3 negative pull-ups<br>1 negative pull-ups<br>1 negative pull-ups<br>up to 2min rest | **8**<br>**10sec** dead hang<br>3 sets in total<br>up to 2min rest | **9**<br>3 negative pull-ups<br>2 negative pull-ups<br>1 negative pull-up<br>up to 2min rest | **10**<br>**10sec** dead hang<br>4 sets in total<br>up to 2min rest |
| **11**<br>3 negative pull-ups<br>2 negative pull-ups<br>2 negative pull-ups<br>up to 2min rest | **12**<br>**10sec** dead hang<br>4 sets in total<br>up to 2min rest | **13**<br>4 negative pull-ups<br>2 negative pull-ups<br>1 negative pull-up<br>up to 2min rest | **14**<br>**15sec** dead hang<br>3 sets in total<br>up to 2min rest | **15**<br>4 negative pull-ups<br>2 negative pull-ups<br>2 negative pull-ups<br>up to 2min rest |
| **16**<br>**15sec** dead hang<br>3 sets in total<br>up to 2min rest | **17**<br>4 negative pull-ups<br>3 negative pull-ups<br>2 negative pull-up<br>up to 2min rest | **18**<br>**15sec** dead hang<br>4 sets in total<br>up to 2min rest | **19**<br>5 negative pull-ups<br>3 negative pull-ups<br>1 negative pull-ups<br>up to 2min rest | **20**<br>**15sec** dead hang<br>4 sets in total<br>up to 2min rest |
| **21**<br>5 negative pull-ups<br>3 negative pull-ups<br>2 negative pull-up<br>up to 2min rest | **22**<br>**20sec** dead hang<br>3 sets in total<br>up to 2min rest | **23**<br>5 negative pull-ups<br>3 negative pull-ups<br>3 negative pull-ups<br>up to 2min rest | **24**<br>**20sec** dead hang<br>3 sets in total<br>up to 2min rest | **25**<br>6 negative pull-ups<br>3 negative pull-ups<br>2 negative pull-ups<br>up to 2min rest |
| **26**<br>**20sec** dead hang<br>4 sets in total<br>up to 2min rest | **27**<br>6 negative pull-ups<br>3 negative pull-ups<br>3 negative pull-ups<br>up to 2min rest | **28**<br>**20sec** dead hang<br>4 sets in total<br>up to 2min rest | **29**<br>6 negative pull-ups<br>4 negative pull-ups<br>3 negative pull-ups<br>up to 2min rest | **30**<br>**30sec** dead hang<br>3 sets in total<br>up to 2min rest |

## 67 Ninja

Let your secret ninja mojo rise this month with the Ninja Challenge. It's designed specifically to take you through each of the many attributes that make a ninja fearsome and effective. A ninja's most fearsome weapon is his mind and though you will be performing mostly physical tasks, each day is intended to take you to a new physical and mental place. Accept the challenge, open yourself to your inner warrior path and remember a ninja is forged from willpower and discipline. All physical change happens because the mind changes first.

# NINJA

## 30-day challenge © darebee.com

Complete the given exercise for each day according to your chosen level, non-stop.

| | |
|---|---|
| normal | **30 seconds** |
| hard | **1 minute** |
| brutal | **2 minutes** |

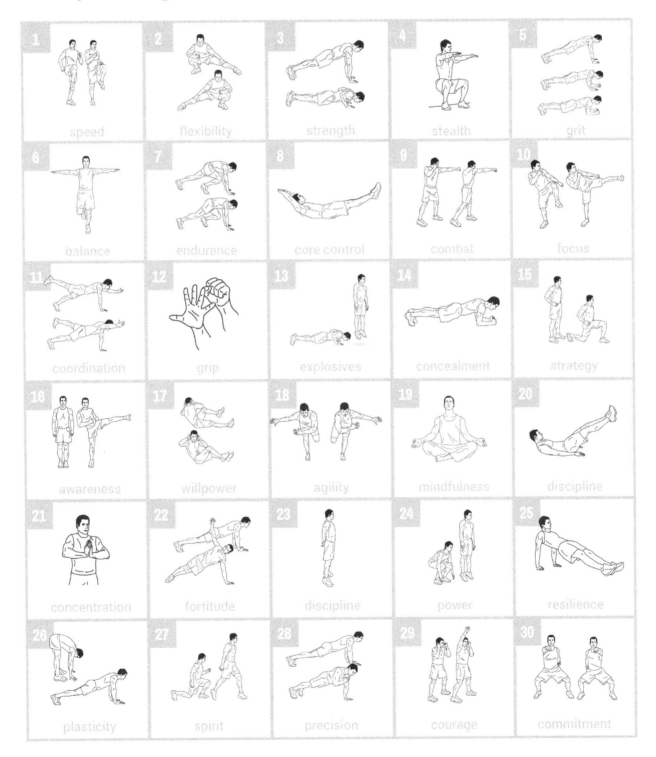

| | | | | |
|---|---|---|---|---|
| 1 speed | 2 flexibility | 3 strength | 4 stealth | 5 grit |
| 6 balance | 7 endurance | 8 core control | 9 combat | 10 focus |
| 11 coordination | 12 grip | 13 explosives | 14 concealment | 15 strategy |
| 16 awareness | 17 willpower | 18 agility | 19 mindfulness | 20 discipline |
| 21 concentration | 22 fortitude | 23 discipline | 24 power | 25 resilience |
| 26 plasticity | 27 spirit | 28 precision | 29 courage | 30 commitment |

## 68   No Junk Food

When it comes to upgrading to a better version of you it is a case of creating small, sustainable changes one day at a time. The No Junk Food Challenge helps you transition from eating habits that undermine your fitness goals and hold you back to a much better approach to nutrition. All you have to do is lay off the junk food for 30 days. You will be surprised how that one small change will affect pretty much everything you do.

# NO JUNK FOOD

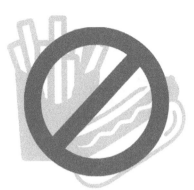

**NO JUNK FOOD FOR 30 DAYS CHALLENGE**

© darebee.com

| | | | | |
|---|---|---|---|---|
| **1** no junk food today! | **2** no junk food today! | **3** no junk food today! | **4** no junk food today! | **5** no junk food today! |
| **6** no junk food today! | **7** no junk food today! | **8** no junk food today! | **9** no junk food today! | **10** no junk food today! |
| **11** no junk food today! | **12** no junk food today! | **13** no junk food today! | **14** no junk food today! | **15** no junk food today! |
| **16** no junk food today! | **17** no junk food today! | **18** no junk food today! | **19** no junk food today! | **20** no junk food today! |
| **21** no junk food today! | **22** no junk food today! | **23** no junk food today! | **24** no junk food today! | **25** no junk food today! |
| **26** no junk food today! | **27** no junk food today! | **28** no junk food today! | **29** no junk food today! | **30** no junk food today! |

## 69 No Salt

If exercise is medicine, food is the very stuff our bodies and minds are made of. What we put in our body affects the way it functions and it affects our mind. Salt is in most foods so each time we add extra salt we are more than likely overdoing it. Going without added salt for 30 days is a great boost to the body's internal functions. It helps it recover from excessive salt processing and reset.

Instructions: Don't add any salt to your food when you serve or cook.

# NO SALT

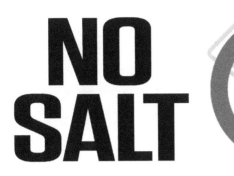

**NO ADDED SALT FOR 30 DAYS CHALLENGE**

© darebee.com

| | | | | |
|---|---|---|---|---|
| **1** No extra salt in my food today! | **2** No extra salt in my food today! | **3** No extra salt in my food today! | **4** No extra salt in my food today! | **5** No extra salt in my food today! |
| **6** No extra salt in my food today! | **7** No extra salt in my food today! | **8** No extra salt in my food today! | **9** No extra salt in my food today! | **10** No extra salt in my food today! |
| **11** No extra salt in my food today! | **12** No extra salt in my food today! | **13** No extra salt in my food today! | **14** No extra salt in my food today! | **15** No extra salt in my food today! |
| **16** No extra salt in my food today! | **17** No extra salt in my food today! | **18** No extra salt in my food today! | **19** No extra salt in my food today! | **20** No extra salt in my food today! |
| **21** No extra salt in my food today! | **22** No extra salt in my food today! | **23** No extra salt in my food today! | **24** No extra salt in my food today! | **25** No extra salt in my food today! |
| **26** No extra salt in my food today! | **27** No extra salt in my food today! | **28** No extra salt in my food today! | **29** No extra salt in my food today! | **30** No extra salt in my food today! |

## 70 No Sugar

Although our taste buds and our body are highly attuned to the pleasure derived from sugar, today there is sugar in many of our foodstuffs and way too much in our diet. This causes problems with our microbiome, it affects our weight and it impacts on our health. The No Sugar challenge helps you address this balance. Over a month, you help your taste buds reset, you aid in the recovery and resetting of your microbiome flora and discover just how much this small dietary change can affect your weight. You build up a new, healthier you by making small changes, one day at a time. This is a good start.

# No Sugar

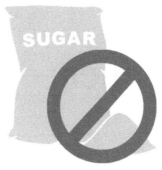

no chocolate,
no cookies,
no soft drinks
for 30 days

© darebee.com

| | | | | |
|---|---|---|---|---|
| **1** no sugar today! | **2** no sugar today! | **3** no sugar today! | **4** no sugar today! | **5** no sugar today! |
| **6** no sugar today! | **7** no sugar today! | **8** no sugar today! | **9** no sugar today! | **10** no sugar today! |
| **11** no sugar today! | **12** no sugar today! | **13** no sugar today! | **14** no sugar today! | **15** no sugar today! |
| **16** no sugar today! | **17** no sugar today! | **18** no sugar today! | **19** no sugar today! | **20** no sugar today! |
| **21** no sugar today! | **22** no sugar today! | **23** no sugar today! | **24** no sugar today! | **25** no sugar today! |
| **26** no sugar today! | **27** no sugar today! | **28** no sugar today! | **29** no sugar today! | **30** no sugar today! |

## 71     Office

Whether you work from home or work in a more traditional office environment, the chances are that you spend a lot of time sitting down and a lot of time trying to earn a living. That doesn't mean your fitness needs to suffer.

Office is a month of daily workouts you can do in an office environment or in the home, if you are working from home. Incrementally, the mini-workouts work their magic, triggering an adaptation response that will physically change you.

# 30-day **office** —challenge—

© darebee.com

| | | | | |
|---|---|---|---|---|
| **1** | **2** | **3** | **4** | **5** |
| **20 seconds** wall-sit | **20 seconds** tricep dip hold | **40 seconds** wall-sit | **40 seconds** tricep dip hold | **60 seconds** wall-sit |
| **6** | **7** | **8** | **9** | **10** |
| **60 seconds** tricep dip hold | **1min 20sec** wall-sit | **1min 20sec** tricep dip hold | **1min 40sec** wall-sit | **1min 40sec** tricep dip hold |
| **11** | **12** | **13** | **14** | **15** |
| **2 minutes** wall-sit | **2 minutes** tricep dip hold | **2min 10sec** wall-sit | **2min 10sec** tricep dip hold | **2min 20sec** wall-sit |
| **16** | **17** | **18** | **19** | **20** |
| **2min 20sec** tricep dip hold | **2min 30sec** wall-sit | **2min 30sec** tricep dip hold | **2min 40sec** wall-sit | **2min 40sec** tricep dip hold |
| **21** | **22** | **23** | **24** | **25** |
| **3 minutes** wall-sit | **3 minutes** tricep dip hold | **3min 10sec** wall-sit | **3min 10sec** tricep dip hold | **3min 20sec** wall-sit |
| **26** | **27** | **28** | **29** | **30** |
| **3min 20sec** tricep dip hold | **3min 30sec** wall-sit | **3min 30sec** tricep dip hold | **4 minutes** wall-sit | **4 minutes** tricep dip hold |

## 72 Only Homemade

We live in times of convenience. Everything we eat nowadays comes in a package and a lot of it is ready to eat. Although buying and eating ready-made meals allows us to focus our time and energy on other things it also lowers the quality of what we fuel our bodies with. After all, no one cares about what goes into our meals more than we do.

Cooking our own food allows us to pick higher quality ingredients, cut back on preservatives and make a lot more nutritious meals. Making things from scratch also helps us better understand what goes into each dish and what we put into our bodies. We really are what we eat and what we digest. We can't hope to build better, healthier and stronger bodies if we don't pay attention to our nutrition.

This challenge calls for 100% homemade meals. It challenges each of us to cook everything we eat from scratch for 30 days. The meals are not required to be complex, low fat, low carb or high protein. You can make anything you want as long as it is made from basic ingredients whether it's soup or bread, salad or muffins. The challenge here is to not rely on anything that comes prepackaged or processed. You can adjust the degree of complexity for this challenge to fit the time available but we recommend making as many things from scratch as possible. For example, try baking your own bread and if you are making beans, use dry beans and not the ones that come from a can. Avoid using any quick mixes or shortcuts altogether during the challenge.

When we make our own food we inevitably increase the nutritional value of every meal. And when our body gets all it needs it stops being in a constant state of distress, our hunger goes down because our nutritional needs are met and we feel more content and satisfied.

# ONLY HOME MADE

**30 DAY CHALLENGE**

EAT ONLY
HOMEMADE
MEALS
FOR 30 DAYS

© darebee.com

| | | | | |
|---|---|---|---|---|
| **1** only homemade meals today | **2** only homemade meals today | **3** only homemade meals today | **4** only homemade meals today | **5** only homemade meals today |
| **6** only homemade meals today | **7** only homemade meals today | **8** only homemade meals today | **9** only homemade meals today | **10** only homemade meals today |
| **11** only homemade meals today | **12** only homemade meals today | **13** only homemade meals today | **14** only homemade meals today | **15** only homemade meals today |
| **16** only homemade meals today | **17** only homemade meals today | **18** only homemade meals today | **19** only homemade meals today | **20** only homemade meals today |
| **21** only homemade meals today | **22** only homemade meals today | **23** only homemade meals today | **24** only homemade meals today | **25** only homemade meals today |
| **26** only homemade meals today | **27** only homemade meals today | **28** only homemade meals today | **29** only homemade meals today | **30** only homemade meals today |

## 73 Plank

The Plank is an exercise that engages many muscles at once. Because the body is locked against the ground it is a closed kinetic chain exercise that loads almost all the abdominal muscle groups, the glutes, the quads, shoulders back and chest. Performed on a daily basis this creates a cumulative, daily physical load that triggers the body's adaptive response.

Planks are a great way to increase overall muscle stability in the body's anterior kinetic chain. This, in turn, improves the body's athleticism.

# PLANK

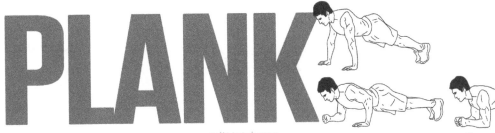

## 30-DAY CHALLENGE

split total reps into manageable sets

© darebee.com

| | | | | |
|---|---|---|---|---|
| **1**<br>10sec plank<br>20sec elbow plank | **2**<br>20sec plank<br>20sec elbow plank | **3**<br>25sec plank<br>20sec elbow plank | **4**<br>5<br>up and down planks | **5**<br>30sec plank<br>20sec elbow plank |
| **6**<br>30sec plank<br>30sec elbow plank | **7**<br>40sec plank<br>30sec elbow plank | **8**<br>10<br>up and down planks | **9**<br>50sec plank<br>30sec elbow plank | **10**<br>1min plank<br>30sec elbow plank |
| **11**<br>1min10sec plank<br>40sec elbow plank | **12**<br>20<br>up and down planks | **13**<br>1min20sec plank<br>40sec elbow plank | **14**<br>1min30sec plank<br>40sec elbow plank | **15**<br>1min40sec plank<br>40sec elbow plank |
| **16**<br>25<br>up and down planks | **17**<br>1min50sec plank<br>45sec elbow plank | **18**<br>2min plank<br>45sec elbow plank | **19**<br>2min10sec plank<br>45sec elbow plank | **20**<br>30<br>up and down planks |
| **21**<br>2min30sec plank<br>50sec elbow plank | **22**<br>2min40sec plank<br>50sec elbow plank | **23**<br>2min50sec plank<br>50sec elbow plank | **24**<br>35<br>up and down planks | **25**<br>3min plank<br>50sec elbow plank |
| **26**<br>3min10sec plank<br>1min elbow plank | **27**<br>3min20sec plank<br>1min elbow plank | **28**<br>40<br>up and down planks | **29**<br>3min30sec plank<br>1min elbow plank | **30**<br>4min plank<br>1min elbow plank |

## 74 Plant Based

Scientific evidence is mounting that plant-based meals reverse aging increase cardiovascular endurance and decrease inflammation markers at a cellular level. They help reduce the amount of damage done by free radicals and unhealthy lifestyle choices. Everything that affects the body systemically, affects the brain. How we age determines how we think and how we feel. This, in turn, affects everything else. The Plant Based Challenge is designed to help you discover how differently your body and brain operate when a cleaner source of fuel is supplied.

Instructions: only eat plant-based meals for 30 days. This means you can't eat meat, dairy and eggs or products containing meat, dairy and eggs. Instead, opt-in for their plant-based alternatives, beans and legumes, fruit and vegetables, mushrooms, nuts and seeds. Replace cows milk with almond, oat or soy milk. If you enjoy yogurts, you can buy their plant-based alternative made from nuts, soy or hemp. There is a huge variety of plant-based cheeses as well if you find yourself missing cheese and crackers. Instead of getting your protein from meat, get it from beans, quinoa, chickpeas, lentils, tofu and tempeh, seitan, nuts and seeds. Some vegetables are also quite high in protein (Calories ratio to protein content) like broccoli and cauliflower.

Once 30 days are up you can judge whether this type of eating is for you and if your health and fitness have improved. Plant-based eating pattern doesn't always agree with everyone but for some it can be life-changing. The only way to find out whether it will work for you is to try.

# 30-DAY CHALLENGE

Only eat plant-based
food for 30 days

© darebee.com

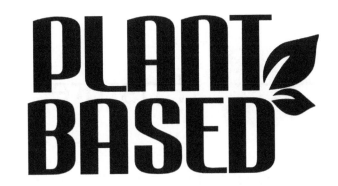

PLANT
BASED

| | | | | |
|---|---|---|---|---|
| **1** Done! | **2** Done! | **3** Done! | **4** Done! | **5** Done! |
| **6** Done! | **7** Done! | **8** Done! | **9** Done! | **10** Done! |
| **11** Done! | **12** Done! | **13** Done! | **14** Done! | **15** Done! |
| **16** Done! | **17** Done! | **18** Done! | **19** Done! | **20** Done! |
| **21** Done! | **22** Done! | **23** Done! | **24** Done! | **25** Done! |
| **26** Done! | **27** Done! | **28** Done! | **29** Done! | **30** Done! |

# 75 Posture

Great posture is made of many different parts which recruit a lot of different muscle groups throughout the body, some of which are required to multi-task in their roles. The Posture Challenge has only two, seemingly simple exercises. To understand how they help improve your posture consider what is required for a good posture to begin with:

- A strong neck and shoulders
- A strong back
- A strong lower back

It is, of course a little more complicated than that as flexibility as well as strength are involved and the front of the body needs to be brought into the picture as well, but the Posture Challenge is simple in what it asks you to do. It targets primarily all the key muscle groups that are not easy to target consistently and by the end of it you will see a difference.

Just so you understand what muscles you are exercising consider that in the neck and upper back consider that anchoring the shoulder blades to the spine is a flat, triangular shaped muscle called the trapezius. This muscle covers the neck, shoulders and thorax. Effective posture necessitates that the trapezius muscle is strengthened equally in the front and back of the body.

On the lower back there are those muscles on the back side of the body which run laterally to the spine, called the erector spinae muscles. Individually, they are the spinalis, longissimus and iliocostalis and they all work together to extend the spine. The multifidus muscles, a smaller group deep in the back, connects the vertebra.

Finally the tail end of the posture support structures are the gluteus and hamstring muscles. Even the hamstrings play a role as they indirectly work to maintain an erect posture during standing and walking.

# office friendly **posture**
## 30-day challenge

© darebee.com

| | | | | |
|---|---|---|---|---|
| **1**<br>**10** side bends<br>repeat twice<br>morning & evening | **2**<br>**20** micro chest expansions<br>**3 sets** in total<br>throughout the day | **3**<br>**12** side bends<br>repeat twice<br>morning & evening | **4**<br>**22** micro chest expansions<br>**3 sets** in total<br>throughout the day | **5**<br>**14** side bends<br>repeat twice<br>morning & evening |
| **6**<br>**24** micro chest expansions<br>**3 sets** in total<br>throughout the day | **7**<br>**16** side bends<br>repeat twice<br>morning & evening | **8**<br>**26** micro chest expansions<br>**3 sets** in total<br>throughout the day | **9**<br>**20** side bends<br>repeat twice<br>morning & evening | **10**<br>**30** micro chest expansions<br>**3 sets** in total<br>throughout the day |
| **11**<br>**22** side bends<br>repeat twice<br>morning & evening | **12**<br>**32** micro chest expansions<br>**3 sets** in total<br>throughout the day | **13**<br>**24** side bends<br>repeat twice<br>morning & evening | **14**<br>**34** micro chest expansions<br>**3 sets** in total<br>throughout the day | **15**<br>**26** side bends<br>repeat twice<br>morning & evening |
| **16**<br>**36** micro chest expansions<br>**3 sets** in total<br>throughout the day | **17**<br>**30** side bends<br>repeat twice<br>morning & evening | **18**<br>**40** micro chest expansions<br>**3 sets** in total<br>throughout the day | **19**<br>**32** side bends<br>repeat twice<br>morning & evening | **20**<br>**42** micro chest expansions<br>**3 sets** in total<br>throughout the day |
| **21**<br>**34** side bends<br>repeat twice<br>morning & evening | **22**<br>**44** micro chest expansions<br>**3 sets** in total<br>throughout the day | **23**<br>**36** side bends<br>repeat twice<br>morning & evening | **24**<br>**46** micro chest expansions<br>**3 sets** in total<br>throughout the day | **25**<br>**40** side bends<br>repeat twice<br>morning & evening |
| **26**<br>**50** micro chest expansions<br>**3 sets** in total<br>throughout the day | **27**<br>**42** side bends<br>repeat twice<br>morning & evening | **28**<br>**52** micro chest expansions<br>**3 sets** in total<br>throughout the day | **29**<br>**44** side bends<br>repeat twice<br>morning & evening | **30**<br>**54** micro chest expansions<br>**3 sets** in total<br>throughout the day |

## 76 Power Grip

The strength of our hand grip is such a reliable measure of upper body strength that it is often used as a measure of overall muscular strength. What is less known perhaps is that a better hand grip strength has been found to be associated with cardiac functions and structures that help reduce the risk of cardiovascular incidents. In addition research indicates that grip strength in midlife can predict physical disability in senior years. All of which mean that you'd better ace this challenge and reap some really long term rewards for it.

Instructions: Clench and unclench your fists as fast and as hard as you can, non-stop, for a given time for each day. Keep up with the animation for maximum results. Clench your fists, tense your arms and hold them over your head to do a flex hold.

# POWER GRIP

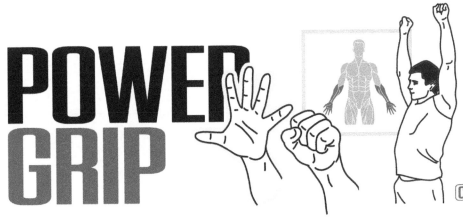

30-day challenge

© darebee.com

| 1 | 2 | 3 | 4 | 5 |
|---|---|---|---|---|
| **40 seconds** clench / unclench | **40 seconds** overhead flex hold | **50 seconds** clench / unclench | **50 seconds** overhead flex hold | **60 seconds** clench / unclench |
| **6** | **7** | **8** | **9** | **10** |
| **60 seconds** overhead flex hold | **1min 10sec** clench / unclench | **1min 10sec** overhead flex hold | **1min 20sec** clench / unclench | **1min 20sec** overhead flex hold |
| **11** | **12** | **13** | **14** | **15** |
| **1min 30sec** clench / unclench | **1min 30sec** overhead flex hold | **1min 40sec** clench / unclench | **1min 40sec** overhead flex hold | **1min 50sec** clench / unclench |
| **16** | **17** | **18** | **19** | **20** |
| **1min 50sec** overhead flex hold | **2 minutes** clench / unclench | **2 minutes** overhead flex hold | **2min 10sec** clench / unclench | **2min 10sec** overhead flex hold |
| **21** | **22** | **23** | **24** | **25** |
| **2min 20sec** clench / unclench | **2min 20sec** overhead flex hold | **2min 30sec** clench / unclench | **2min 30sec** overhead flex hold | **2min 40sec** clench / unclench |
| **26** | **27** | **28** | **29** | **30** |
| **2min 40sec** overhead flex hold | **2min 50sec** clench / unclench | **2min 50sec** overhead flex hold | **3 minutes** clench / unclench | **3 minutes** overhead flex hold |

# 77    Power Pull

Get your upper body and core chiseled with this 15-day pull-up bar challenge. It is beginner-friendly so, as long as you access to a pull-up bar, you can take it up! The rules are simple: hit the given amount of reps by splitting the total into as many sets and taking as much rest as you need. Make it challenging - do as fewer sets as you possibly can. 2 Minutes rest between sets is the recommended rest time.

On core days while doing knee-ins with twists make sure you tighten up your abs and bring your knees up as high as you can to get the most out of the exercise. Can't do twists just yet? Start by bringing your knees up without a twist first until you feel confident you can add the twisting motion.

# Power Pull

CHALLENGE © darebee.com

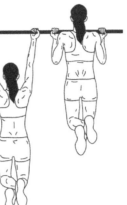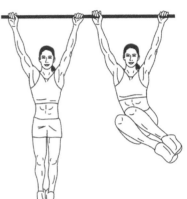

split the goal total
into manageable sets -
as few as possible

| 1 | 2 | 3 | 4 | 5 |
|---|---|---|---|---|
| **to failure** chin-ups<br>**goal** 8 in total | **8** knee-up twists<br>3 sets in total<br>2 minutes rest | **to failure** chin-ups<br>**goal** 8 in total | **8** knee-up twists<br>3 sets in total<br>2 minutes rest | **to failure** chin-ups<br>**goal** 10 in total |
| **6** | **7** | **8** | **9** | **10** |
| **10** knee-up twists<br>3 sets in total<br>2 minutes rest | **to failure** chin-ups<br>**goal** 10 in total | **10** knee-up twists<br>3 sets in total<br>2 minutes rest | **to failure** chin-ups<br>**goal** 12 in total | **12** knee-up twists<br>3 sets in total<br>2 minutes rest |
| **11** | **12** | **13** | **14** | **15** |
| **to failure** chin-ups<br>**goal** 12 in total | **12** knee-up twists<br>3 sets in total<br>2 minutes rest | **to failure** chin-ups<br>**goal** 14 in total | **14** knee-up twists<br>3 sets in total<br>2 minutes rest | **to failure** chin-ups<br>**goal** 14 in total |

## 78 Power Walk

Walking is a great way to raise your body's temperature without breaking into a sweat. It is a great, low-impact exercise that gets your cardiovascular system going and gently increases your metabolic burn. Done on a daily basis it is a great way to lower your resting heart rate, improve your fitness and increase your overall baseline for physical activity.

Set the time and Go! Make sure you bring your knees up and move your arms, as illustrated, for a proper power walk. Every other day all you need to do is power walk for 2 minutes. The challenge is to keep it up!

# power walk
## 30-day challenge

© darebee.com

| | | | | |
|---|---|---|---|---|
| **1**<br>**2 minutes**<br>march steps | **2**<br>**3 minutes**<br>march steps | **3**<br>**2 minutes**<br>march steps | **4**<br>**3min 30sec**<br>march steps | **5**<br>**2 minutes**<br>march steps |
| **6**<br>**4 minutes**<br>march steps | **7**<br>**2 minutes**<br>march steps | **8**<br>**4 min 30sec**<br>march steps | **9**<br>**2 minutes**<br>march steps | **10**<br>**5 minutes**<br>march steps |
| **11**<br>**2 minutes**<br>march steps | **12**<br>**5 min 30sec**<br>march steps | **13**<br>**2 minutes**<br>march steps | **14**<br>**6 minutes**<br>march steps | **15**<br>**2 minutes**<br>march steps |
| **16**<br>**6 min 30sec**<br>march steps | **17**<br>**2 minutes**<br>march steps | **18**<br>**7 minutes**<br>march steps | **19**<br>**2 minutes**<br>march steps | **20**<br>**7 min 30sec**<br>march steps |
| **21**<br>**2 minutes**<br>march steps | **22**<br>**8 minutes**<br>march steps | **23**<br>**2 minutes**<br>march steps | **24**<br>**8 min 30sec**<br>march steps | **25**<br>**2 minutes**<br>march steps |
| **26**<br>**9 minutes**<br>march steps | **27**<br>**2 minutes**<br>march steps | **28**<br>**9min 30sec**<br>march steps | **29**<br>**2 minutes**<br>march steps | **30**<br>**10 minutes**<br>march steps |

# 79 Pull-Up

Defying gravity helps the body develop excellent fuctional strength. Nothing defies gravity quite the way a pull-up does. Over 30 days you get to develop your upper body strength, fascial fitness, upper back and neck, chest and arms and shoulders. It also works the abs and core a little.

Pull-ups are an excellent means of developing the kind of functional upper body strength favored by boxers, gymnasts and martial artists.

# pull-up

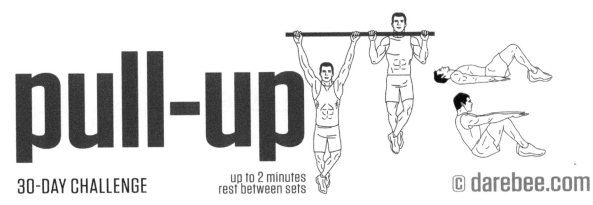

**30-DAY CHALLENGE**

up to 2 minutes
rest between sets

© darebee.com

| | | | | |
|---|---|---|---|---|
| **1**<br>1 pull-up<br>1 pull-up<br>1 pull-up | **2**<br>10 sit-ups<br>3 sets | **3**<br>2 pull-ups<br>1 pull-up<br>1 pull-up | **4**<br>10 sit-ups<br>3 sets | **5**<br>2 pull-ups<br>2 pull-ups<br>1 pull-up |
| **6**<br>15 sit-ups<br>3 sets | **7**<br>2 pull-ups<br>2 pull-ups<br>2 pull-ups | **8**<br>15 sit-ups<br>3 sets | **9**<br>3 pull-ups<br>2 pull-ups<br>1 pull-up | **10**<br>15 sit-ups<br>3 sets |
| **11**<br>3 pull-ups<br>2 pull-ups<br>2 pull-ups | **12**<br>15 sit-ups<br>4 sets | **13**<br>4 pull-ups<br>2 pull-ups<br>1 pull-up | **14**<br>15 sit-ups<br>4 sets | **15**<br>4 pull-ups<br>2 pull-ups<br>2 pull-ups |
| **16**<br>20 sit-ups<br>4 sets | **17**<br>5 pull-ups<br>3 pull-ups<br>1 pull-up | **18**<br>20 sit-ups<br>4 sets | **19**<br>5 pull-ups<br>4 pull-ups<br>2 pull-ups | **20**<br>20 sit-ups<br>4 sets |
| **21**<br>6 pull-ups<br>4 pull-ups<br>1 pull-up | **22**<br>20 sit-ups<br>5 sets | **23**<br>7 pull-ups<br>4 pull-ups<br>2 pull-ups | **24**<br>20 sit-ups<br>5 sets 5 sets | **25**<br>8 pull-ups<br>4 pull-ups<br>3 pull-ups |
| **26**<br>20 sit-ups<br>6 sets | **27**<br>9 pull-ups<br>4 pull-ups<br>2 pull-ups | **28**<br>20 sit-ups<br>6 sets | **29**<br>rest day | **30**<br>10 pull-ups<br>5 pull-ups<br>3 pull-ups |

## 80 Pull-Up Level 2

Pull-ups are difficult because of the physics involved in the equation. Basically the work your arms have to do is described as the energy needed to move some mass over some distance. In the case of doing a single pull-up, the work that your arms and back need to do is a function of your mass and how far you need to move it upwards to get your chin over the bar.

This lets you understand just what an achievement doing pull-ups is and why there is so much value in the bragging rights. This challenge takes you several levels up.

# pull-up

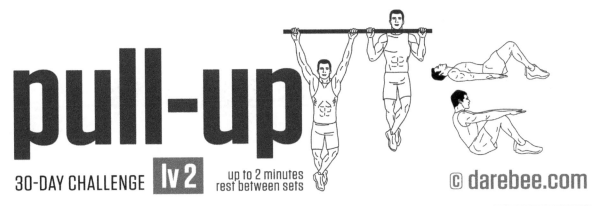

**30-DAY CHALLENGE** **lv 2**   up to 2 minutes
rest between sets   © **darebee.com**

| | | | | |
|---|---|---|---|---|
| **1**<br>10 pull-ups<br>6 pull-ups<br>4 pull-ups | **2**<br>20 sit-ups<br>3 sets<br>twice a day | **3**<br>10 pull-ups<br>8 pull-ups<br>6 pull-ups | **4**<br>20 sit-ups<br>3 sets<br>twice a day | **5**<br>12 pull-ups<br>8 pull-ups<br>4 pull-ups |
| **6**<br>25 sit-ups<br>3 sets<br>twice a day | **7**<br>14 pull-ups<br>6 pull-ups<br>2 pull-ups | **8**<br>25 sit-ups<br>3 sets<br>twice a day | **9**<br>14 pull-ups<br>8 pull-ups<br>2 pull-ups | **10**<br>25 sit-ups<br>3 sets<br>twice a day |
| **11**<br>15 pull-ups<br>6 pull-ups<br>2 pull-ups | **12**<br>20 sit-ups<br>4 sets<br>twice a day | **13**<br>15 pull-ups<br>8 pull-ups<br>2 pull-ups | **14**<br>20 sit-ups<br>4 sets<br>twice a day | **15**<br>16 pull-ups<br>6 pull-ups<br>2 pull-ups |
| **16**<br>20 sit-ups<br>3 sets<br>three times a day | **17**<br>16 pull-ups<br>6 pull-ups<br>4 pull-ups | **18**<br>20 sit-ups<br>3 sets<br>three times a day | **19**<br>17 pull-ups<br>6 pull-ups<br>2 pull-ups | **20**<br>20 sit-ups<br>3 sets<br>three times a day |
| **21**<br>17 pull-ups<br>6 pull-ups<br>4 pull-ups | **22**<br>20 sit-ups<br>4 sets<br>three times a day | **23**<br>17 pull-ups<br>8 pull-ups<br>2 pull-ups | **24**<br>20 sit-ups<br>4 sets<br>three times a day | **25**<br>18 pull-ups<br>8 pull-ups<br>4 pull-ups |
| **26**<br>20 sit-ups<br>3 sets<br>four times a day | **27**<br>19 pull-ups<br>8 pull-ups<br>4 pull-ups | **28**<br>20 sit-ups<br>3 sets<br>four times a day | **29**<br>rest day | **30**<br>20 pull-ups<br>8 pull-ups<br>6 pull-ups |

## 81 Punches & Squats

Legs and arms are the natural extensions of the body's ability to generate power. Using them correctly requires specific exercises that help build strength and coordination. The Punches & Squats, 30-day Challenge appears to be simple yet it effectively targets the crucial muscle groups involved and forces them to build the neural connections necessary for coordinating them better. By the end of the 30-Day Challenge you will feel and move differently.

# PUNCHES & SQUATS

## 30-DAY CHALLENGE

© darebee.com

| 1 | 2 | 3 | 4 | 5 |
|---|---|---|---|---|
| **30** punches<br>3 sets in total<br>30sec rest | **50** squats<br>in total<br>throughout the day | **30** punches<br>3 sets in total<br>30sec rest | **55** squats<br>in total<br>throughout the day | **40** punches<br>3 sets in total<br>30sec rest |
| 6 | 7 | 8 | 9 | 10 |
| **60** squats<br>in total<br>throughout the day | **40** punches<br>3 sets in total<br>30sec rest | **65** squats<br>in total<br>throughout the day | **50** punches<br>3 sets in total<br>30sec rest | **70** squats<br>in total<br>throughout the day |
| 11 | 12 | 13 | 14 | 15 |
| **50** punches<br>3 sets in total<br>30sec rest | **75** squats<br>in total<br>throughout the day | **60** punches<br>3 sets in total<br>30sec rest | **80** squats<br>in total<br>throughout the day | **60** punches<br>3 sets in total<br>30sec rest |
| 16 | 17 | 18 | 19 | 20 |
| **85** squats<br>in total<br>throughout the day | **70** punches<br>3 sets in total<br>30sec rest | **90** squats<br>in total<br>throughout the day | **70** punches<br>3 sets in total<br>30sec rest | **95** squats<br>in total<br>throughout the day |
| 21 | 22 | 23 | 24 | 25 |
| **80** punches<br>3 sets in total<br>30sec rest | **100** squats<br>in total<br>throughout the day | **80** punches<br>3 sets in total<br>30sec rest | **105** squats<br>in total<br>throughout the day | **90** punches<br>3 sets in total<br>30sec rest |
| 26 | 27 | 28 | 29 | 30 |
| **110** squats<br>in total<br>throughout the day | **90** punches<br>3 sets in total<br>30sec rest | **115** squats<br>in total<br>throughout the day | **100** punches<br>3 sets in total<br>30sec rest | **120** squats<br>in total<br>throughout the day |

## 82 Punch Out

Channel your angst, inner anguish and deepest frustrations into an upper body, daily, workout that will transform how you feel; change how you move and totally make you feel better about yourself inside and out. The Punch Out! Challenge will help you pile up the numbers. In addition this will help your cardiovascular and aerobic fitness, help decrease your resting heartbeat, increase your base metabolic rate. It will also help increase your upper limb speed which is no bad thing either.

# PUNCH OUT!

## 30-DAY CHALLENGE

© darebee.com

| | | | | |
|---|---|---|---|---|
| **1**<br>**80**<br>punches | **2**<br>**80**<br>overhead punches | **3**<br>**120**<br>punches | **4**<br>**120**<br>overhead punches | **5**<br>**140**<br>punches |
| **6**<br>**140**<br>overhead punches | **7**<br>**160**<br>punches | **8**<br>**160**<br>overhead punches | **9**<br>**200**<br>punches | **10**<br>**200**<br>overhead punches |
| **11**<br>**240**<br>punches | **12**<br>**240**<br>overhead punches | **13**<br>**260**<br>punches | **14**<br>**260**<br>overhead punches | **15**<br>**300**<br>punches |
| **16**<br>**300**<br>overhead punches | **17**<br>**340**<br>punches | **18**<br>**340**<br>overhead punches | **19**<br>**380**<br>punches | **20**<br>**380**<br>overhead punches |
| **21**<br>**400**<br>punches | **22**<br>**400**<br>overhead punches | **23**<br>**420**<br>punches | **24**<br>**420**<br>overhead punches | **25**<br>**460**<br>punches |
| **26**<br>**460**<br>overhead punches | **27**<br>**480**<br>punches | **28**<br>**480**<br>overhead punches | **29**<br>**500**<br>punches | **30**<br>**500**<br>overhead punches |

## 83 Push-Up Ladder

The Push-Up Ladder challenge focuses on your upper body: triceps, biceps, chest, back, abs and core. Push-up focused days will gradually take you to a more advanced push-up style that will give you increased upper body strength and more control over your body. Punching days engage the same muscles but in a less direct way helping you recover while keeping up the focus. The closer punching sets are performed to each other the better but the total can be comfortably split and spread throughout the day. One set of the ladder (wide grip, classic grip and close grip) is performed without rest between exercises - you switch on the fly.

This challenge can be scaled down to fit your fitness level:
Do only one set of the ladder for Level I.
Two sets of the ladder for Level II.
Do all three sets of the ladder for level III.

The challenge is designed for performance and visual results.

# push-up ladder

## 30-DAY CHALLENGE

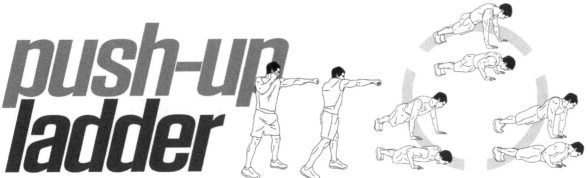

© darebee.com

| 1 | 2 | 3 | 4 | 5 |
|---|---|---|---|---|
| 4 wide grip<br>6 classic grip<br>4 close grip<br>30sec rest \| 3 sets | **500** punches throughout the day | 4 wide grip<br>8 classic grip<br>4 close grip<br>30sec rest \| 3 sets | **500** punches throughout the day | 4 wide grip<br>10 classic grip<br>4 close grip<br>30sec rest \| 3 sets |
| **6** | **7** | **8** | **9** | **10** |
| **600** punches throughout the day | 4 wide grip<br>12 classic grip<br>4 close grip<br>30sec rest \| 3 sets | **600** punches throughout the day | 4 wide grip<br>14 classic grip<br>4 close grip<br>30sec rest \| 3 sets | **700** punches throughout the day |
| **11** | **12** | **13** | **14** | **15** |
| 6 wide grip<br>4 classic grip<br>4 close grip<br>30sec rest \| 3 sets | **700** punches throughout the day | 8 wide grip<br>4 classic grip<br>4 close grip<br>30sec rest \| 3 sets | **800** punches throughout the day | 10 wide grip<br>4 classic grip<br>4 close grip<br>30sec rest \| 3 sets |
| **16** | **17** | **18** | **19** | **20** |
| **800** punches throughout the day | 12 wide grip<br>4 classic grip<br>4 close grip<br>30sec rest \| 3 sets | **900** punches throughout the day | 14 wide grip<br>4 classic grip<br>4 close grip<br>30sec rest \| 3 sets | **900** punches throughout the day |
| **21** | **22** | **23** | **24** | **25** |
| 4 wide grip<br>4 classic grip<br>6 close grip<br>30sec rest \| 3 sets | **1000** punches throughout the day | 4 wide grip<br>4 classic grip<br>8 close grip<br>30sec rest \| 3 sets | **1000** punches throughout the day | 4 wide grip<br>4 classic grip<br>10 close grip<br>30sec rest \| 3 sets |
| **26** | **27** | **28** | **29** | **30** |
| **1200** punches throughout the day | 4 wide grip<br>4 classic grip<br>12 close grip<br>30sec rest \| 3 sets | **1200** punches throughout the day | 4 wide grip<br>4 classic grip<br>14 close grip<br>30sec rest \| 3 sets | **1400** punches throughout the day |

## 84 Push-Up Master

Push-ups are a closed kinetic chain exercise that pit the body's strength against the pull of the planet's gravity well. As such they engage virtually all the muscles and tendons of the body's front kinetic change and also engage the glutes, lower back and core. This is why they are such an intensive exercise. At the same time they deliver excellent physical fitness results.

Extra Credit: Complete the total reps for your level in one go.

# push-up master

## 30-Day Challenge © darebee.com

Pick a level and complete
the given number & style
of push-ups every day for 30 days.

easy      **10 push-ups**
hard      **20 push-ups**
advanced  **30 push-ups**

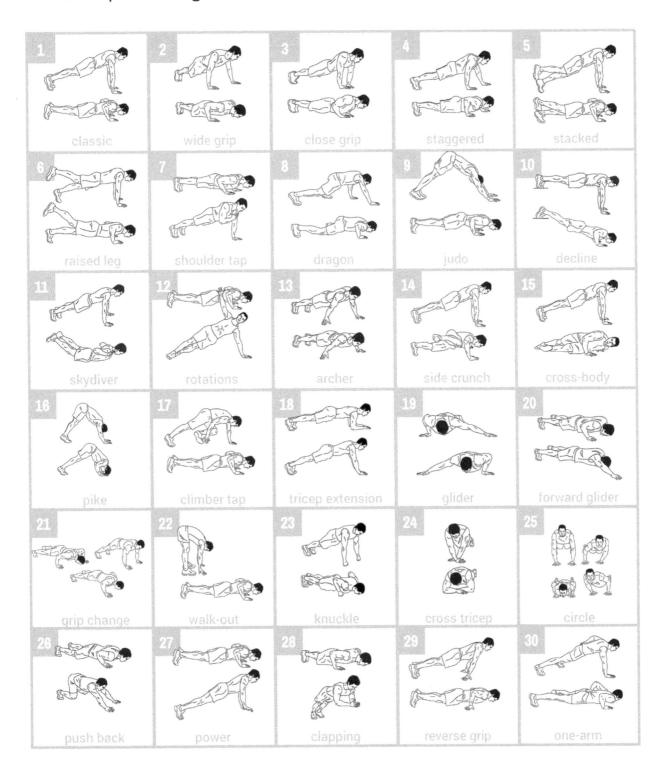

| | | | | |
|---|---|---|---|---|
| 1 classic | 2 wide grip | 3 close grip | 4 staggered | 5 stacked |
| 6 raised leg | 7 shoulder tap | 8 dragon | 9 judo | 10 decline |
| 11 skydiver | 12 rotations | 13 archer | 14 side crunch | 15 cross-body |
| 16 pike | 17 climber tap | 18 tricep extension | 19 glider | 20 forward glider |
| 21 grip change | 22 walk-out | 23 knuckle | 24 cross tricep | 25 circle |
| 26 push back | 27 power | 28 clapping | 29 reverse grip | 30 one-arm |

## 85    Salad A Day

Eating a salad a day is a good way to add more veggies into our daily menu. Adding vegetables to our diet is good for the health of our gut and the flora that lives there and it also affects the way our body regulates the energy we get from food. Developing the good habit of eating a salad a day however requires some practice. By committing to the challenge we develop eating habits that will be beneficial to your fitness and health.

# A SALAD A DAY

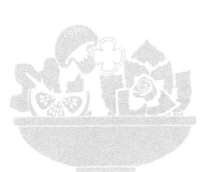

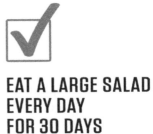

**EAT A LARGE SALAD EVERY DAY FOR 30 DAYS**

© darebee.com

| | | | | |
|---|---|---|---|---|
| **1** I ate a salad today! | **2** I ate a salad today! | **3** I ate a salad today! | **4** I ate a salad today! | **5** I ate a salad today! |
| **6** I ate a salad today! | **7** I ate a salad today! | **8** I ate a salad today! | **9** I ate a salad today! | **10** I ate a salad today! |
| **11** I ate a salad today! | **12** I ate a salad today! | **13** I ate a salad today! | **14** I ate a salad today! | **15** I ate a salad today! |
| **16** I ate a salad today! | **17** I ate a salad today! | **18** I ate a salad today! | **19** I ate a salad today! | **20** I ate a salad today! |
| **21** I ate a salad today! | **22** I ate a salad today! | **23** I ate a salad today! | **24** I ate a salad today! | **25** I ate a salad today! |
| **26** I ate a salad today! | **27** I ate a salad today! | **28** I ate a salad today! | **29** I ate a salad today! | **30** I ate a salad today! |

## 86 Spartan

When you think about Spartan training you have to consider whole body training. The Spartans are the perfect example of early "special forces". Their devotion to training stood at the core of their lifestyle. As a result they left nothing to chance. Spartan is a challenge that asks you to train your entire body, in small ways, over a month. In return you will see and feel real changes take place that will form the basis for your leveling up in your fitness level.

# SPARTAN
## 30-DAY CHALLENGE

© darebee.com

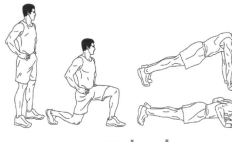

| | | | | |
|---|---|---|---|---|
| **1**<br>**40** punches<br>3 sets in total<br>20sec rest | **2**<br>**40 seconds**<br>one-arm plank<br>in one go | **3**<br>**10** lunges<br>3 sets in total<br>20sec rest | **4**<br>**40** punches<br>4 sets in total<br>20sec rest | **5**<br>**40 seconds**<br>one-arm plank<br>in one go |
| **6**<br>**10** lunges<br>4 sets in total<br>20sec rest | **7**<br>**60** punches<br>3 sets in total<br>20sec rest | **8**<br>**1 minute**<br>one-arm plank<br>in one go | **9**<br>**14** lunges<br>3 sets in total<br>20sec rest | **10**<br>**60** punches<br>4 sets in total<br>20sec rest |
| **11**<br>**1 minute**<br>one-arm plank<br>in one go | **12**<br>**14** lunges<br>4 sets in total<br>20sec rest | **13**<br>**80** punches<br>3 sets in total<br>20sec rest | **14**<br>**1min 20sec**<br>one-arm plank<br>in one go | **15**<br>**18** lunges<br>3 sets in total<br>20sec rest |
| **16**<br>**80** punches<br>4 sets in total<br>20sec rest | **17**<br>**1min 20sec**<br>one-arm plank<br>in one go | **18**<br>**18** lunges<br>4 sets in total<br>20sec rest | **19**<br>**100** punches<br>3 sets in total<br>20sec rest | **20**<br>**1min 40sec**<br>one-arm plank<br>in one go |
| **21**<br>**20** lunges<br>3 sets in total<br>20sec rest | **22**<br>**100** punches<br>4 sets in total<br>20sec rest | **23**<br>**1min 40sec**<br>one-arm plank<br>in one go | **24**<br>**20** lunges<br>4 sets in total<br>20sec rest | **25**<br>**120** punches<br>3 sets in total<br>20sec rest |
| **26**<br>**2 minutes**<br>one-arm plank<br>in one go | **27**<br>**22** lunges<br>3 sets in total<br>20sec rest | **28**<br>**120** punches<br>4 sets in total<br>20sec rest | **29**<br>**2 minutes**<br>one-arm plank<br>in one go | **30**<br>**22** lunges<br>4 sets in total<br>20sec rest |

## 87 Splits

Flexibility is the key to unleashing power and speed by increasing the range of motion active (agonist) muscles have to travel before they are held back by the opposing (antagonist) ones. Being more flexible can also reduce the chances of injury when exercising, though the biggest benefit will be in the way you walk and stand. This 30-day program will help you increase your flexibility. The program utilizes a mixture of active (leg raises) and passive (holding the splits position) stretching techniques to give you the fastest gains possible in the shortest time.

Tip: it will help if you also do long distance running. Do the side splits right after the run when your muscles are all warmed up.

# splits

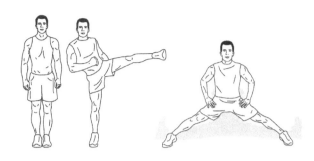

## 30-DAY CHALLENGE

split total reps into manageable sets

© darebee.com

| | | | | |
|---|---|---|---|---|
| **1**<br>40 leg raises<br>40sec side splits | **2**<br>60 leg raises<br>1min side splits | **3**<br>80 leg raises<br>1min20sec side splits | **4**<br>100 leg raises<br>1min40sec side splits | **5**<br>120 leg raises<br>2min side splits |
| **6**<br>140 leg raises<br>2min20sec side splits | **7**<br>160 leg raises<br>2min40sec side splits | **8**<br>180 leg raises<br>3min side splits | **9**<br>200 leg raises<br>3min20sec side splits | **10**<br>220 leg raises<br>3min40sec side splits |
| **11**<br>240 leg raises<br>4min side splits | **12**<br>260 leg raises<br>4min20sec side splits | **13**<br>280 leg raises<br>4min40sec side splits | **14**<br>300 leg raises<br>5min side splits | **15**<br>320 leg raises<br>5min20sec side splits |
| **16**<br>340 leg raises<br>5min40sec side splits | **17**<br>360 leg raises<br>6min side splits | **18**<br>380 leg raises<br>6min20sec side splits | **19**<br>400 leg raises<br>6min40sec side splits | **20**<br>420 leg raises<br>7min side splits |
| **21**<br>440 leg raises<br>7min20sec side splits | **22**<br>460 leg raises<br>7min40sec side splits | **23**<br>480 leg raises<br>8min side splits | **24**<br>500 leg raises<br>8min20sec side splits | **25**<br>520 leg raises<br>8min40sec side splits |
| **26**<br>540 leg raises<br>9min side splits | **27**<br>560 leg raises<br>9min20sec side splits | **28**<br>580 leg raises<br>9min30sec side splits | **29**<br>600 leg raises<br>9min40sec side splits | **30**<br>620 leg raises<br>10min side splits |

## 88 Squats & Punches

Squats and punches train both the lower and upper kinetic chains of the body. Squats are the perfect closed chain lower body kinetic exercise while punches are an open upper body kinetic chain exercise. The result is a variable load that is distributed on the muscles as you progress from day to day. This, in turn, activates the body's adaptive response to produce, over a month, physical changes that help you become healthier, stronger and in greater control of the body you live in.

# 30-DAY-CHALLENGE
# SQUATS
## & punches

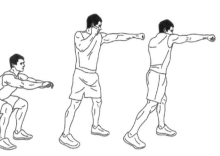

© darebee.com

**1**
**20**
squats
3 sets | 20sec rest

**2**
**20**
jab + cross + squat
3 sets | 20sec rest

**3**
**250**
punches
in total for the day

**4**
**22**
squats
3 sets | 20sec rest

**5**
**22**
jab + cross + squat
3 sets | 20sec rest

**6**
**300**
punches
in total for the day

**7**
**24**
squats
3 sets | 20sec rest

**8**
**24**
jab + cross + squat
3 sets | 20sec rest

**9**
**350**
punches
in total for the day

**10**
**20**
squats
4 sets | 20sec rest

**11**
**20**
jab + cross + squat
4 sets | 20sec rest

**12**
**400**
punches
in total for the day

**13**
**22**
squats
4 sets | 20sec rest

**14**
**22**
jab + cross + squat
4 sets | 20sec rest

**15**
**450**
punches
in total for the day

**16**
**24**
squats
4 sets | 20sec rest

**17**
**24**
jab + cross + squat
4 sets | 20sec rest

**18**
**500**
punches
in total for the day

**19**
**20**
squats
5 sets | 20sec rest

**20**
**20**
jab + cross + squat
5 sets | 20sec rest

**21**
**550**
punches
in total for the day

**22**
**22**
squats
5 sets | 20sec rest

**23**
**22**
jab + cross + squat
5 sets | 20sec rest

**24**
**600**
punches
in total for the day

**25**
**24**
squats
5 sets | 20sec rest

**26**
**24**
jab + cross + squat
5 sets | 20sec rest

**27**
**650**
punches
in total for the day

**28**
**26**
squats
5 sets | 20sec rest

**29**
**26**
jab + cross + squat
5 sets | 20sec rest

**30**
**700**
punches
in total for the day

## 89 Squats

Quads are the largest muscle in the body by muscle mass. As a result exercising them is great for the cardiovascular and aerobic systems. As they get stronger they make the body feel lighter. Getting about on foot becomes a breeze. Your running and jumping will definitely improve but you will also find that you tire less. The biggest benefit by far however is that squats also increase the level of power your body can generate. Everything, from punching to lifting becomes that much easier.

Level I: 30 seconds rest between sets
Level II: 20 seconds rest between sets
Level III: 10 seconds rest between sets

# SQUATS

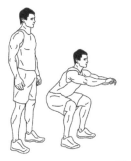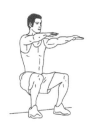

**30-DAY CHALLENGE**

© darebee.com

| | | | | |
|---|---|---|---|---|
| **1**<br>10 squats<br>6 squats<br>6 squats | **2**<br>16 squats<br>10 squats<br>10 squats | **3**<br>18 squats<br>10 squats<br>10 squats | **4**<br>30sec<br>wall sit | **5**<br>20 squats<br>6 squats<br>6 squats |
| **6**<br>22 squats<br>6 squats<br>6 squats | **7**<br>24 squats<br>10 squats<br>10 squats | **8**<br>40sec<br>wall sit | **9**<br>26 squats<br>10 squats<br>10 squats | **10**<br>28 squats<br>6 squats<br>6 squats |
| **11**<br>30 squats<br>6 squats<br>6 squats | **12**<br>1min<br>wall sit | **13**<br>32 squats<br>10 squats<br>10 squats | **14**<br>34 squats<br>10 squats<br>10 squats | **15**<br>36 squats<br>10 squats<br>10 squats |
| **16**<br>1min 20sec<br>wall sit | **17**<br>38 squats<br>6 squats<br>6 squats | **18**<br>40 squats<br>10 squats<br>10 squats | **19**<br>42 squats<br>10 squats<br>10 squats | **20**<br>1min 40sec<br>wall sit |
| **21**<br>44 squats<br>6 squats<br>6 squats | **22**<br>46 squats<br>6 squats<br>6 squats | **23**<br>48 squats<br>10 squats<br>10 squats | **24**<br>2 min<br>wall sit | **25**<br>50 squats<br>10 squats<br>10 squats |
| **26**<br>52 squats<br>6 squats<br>6 squats | **27**<br>54 squats<br>6 squats<br>6 squats | **28**<br>2min 20sec<br>wall sit | **29**<br>56 squats<br>10 squats<br>10 squats | **30**<br>60 squats<br>20 squats<br>20 squats |

# 90 Squats & Push-Ups

Nothing is impossible provided you take a structured approach to it. This is exactly what it is and if doing 3,000 squats and 1,000 push-ups sounds impossible, this workout shows just how it can be done. Doing it helps bolster your confidence in your own abilities, dedication, discipline and commitment. Plus it just totally feels good to see the numbers add up.

# 3,000 squats
# 1,000 push-ups

**30-DAY CHALLENGE**   split total reps into manageable sets

© darebee.com

| | | | | |
|---|---|---|---|---|
| **1** 100 squats | **2** 20 push-ups | **3** 120 squats | **4** 40 push-ups | **5** 140 squats |
| **6** 40 push-ups | **7** 150 squats | **8** 50 push-ups | **9** 160 squats | **10** 50 push-ups |
| **11** 170 squats | **12** 60 push-ups | **13** 180 squats | **14** 60 push-ups | **15** 200 squats |
| **16** 70 push-ups | **17** 220 squats | **18** 70 push-ups | **19** 230 squats | **20** 80 push-ups |
| **21** 240 squats | **22** 80 push-ups | **23** 250 squats | **24** 90 push-ups | **25** 260 squats |
| **26** 90 push-ups | **27** 280 squats | **28** 100 push-ups | **29** 300 squats | **30** 100 push-ups |

## 91    Target 10

Target 10 gives you the opportunity to excel at doing ten distinct exercises through incremental, daily practice over a month. From one day to the next you will add to a cumulative load that will challenge your body to adapt and respond, increasing your control over it. Owning the body you live in takes time, patience and perseverance. Target 10 is a good start on that path.

# TARGET 10

10 MINUTES A DAY. FOR 30 DAYS.

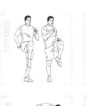     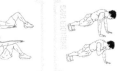

© darebee.com

| | | | | |
|---|---|---|---|---|
| **1**<br>1min high knees<br>1min jumping jacks<br>1min rest \| 5 sets | **2**<br>20sec squats<br>20sec sit-ups<br>20sec squats<br>1min rest \| 10 sets | **3**<br>10 minutes<br>punches<br>non-stop | **4**<br>40sec squats<br>20sec shoulder taps<br>1min rest \| 7 sets<br>finish: 3min squats | **5**<br>20sec high knees<br>20sec climbers<br>20sec high knees<br>1min rest \| 10 sets |
| **6**<br>1min sit-ups<br>1min flutter kicks<br>2min rest \| 5 sets | **7**<br>10 minutes<br>side-to-side<br>leg raises<br>non-stop | **8**<br>30sec jumping jacks<br>30sec plank jacks<br>1min rest \| 7 sets<br>finish: 3min jacks | **9**<br>20sec squats<br>20sec punches<br>20sec squats<br>1min rest \| 10 sets | **10**<br>1min climbers<br>1min flutter kicks<br>2min rest \| 5 sets |
| **11**<br>10 minutes<br>punches<br>non-stop | **12**<br>20sec high knees<br>20sec jumping jacks<br>20sec high knees<br>1min rest \| 10 sets | **13**<br>30sec punches<br>30sec shoulder taps<br>1min rest \| 7 sets<br>finish: 3min punches | **14**<br>1min squats<br>1min flutter kicks<br>2min rest \| 5 sets | **15**<br>10 minutes<br>side-to-side<br>leg raises<br>non-stop |
| **16**<br>1min jumping jacks<br>1min punches<br>2min rest \| 4 sets<br>finish: 2min sit-ups | **17**<br>20sec high knees<br>20sec climbers<br>20sec high knees<br>1min rest \| 10 sets | **18**<br>40sec squats<br>20sec shoulder taps<br>1min rest \| 7 sets<br>finish: 3min squats | **19**<br>10 minutes<br>punches<br>non-stop | **20**<br>30sec high knees<br>30sec climbers<br>30sec high knees<br>30sec plank jacks<br>2min rest \| 5 sets |
| **21**<br>20sec squats<br>20sec sit-ups<br>20sec flutter kicks<br>1min rest \| 10 sets | **22**<br>1min jumping jacks<br>1min high knees<br>2min rest \| 4 sets<br>finish: 2min climbers | **23**<br>10 minutes<br>side-to-side<br>leg raises<br>non-stop | **24**<br>40sec squats<br>20sec shoulder taps<br>1min rest \| 7 sets<br>finish: 3min squats | **25**<br>1min jumping jacks<br>1min rest \| 10 sets |
| **26**<br>30sec high knees<br>30sec flutter kicks<br>30sec high knees<br>30sec sit-ups<br>2min rest \| 5 sets | **27**<br>10 minutes<br>punches<br>non-stop | **28**<br>40sec punches<br>20sec shoulder taps<br>1min rest \| 7 sets<br>finish: 3min punches | **29**<br>1min sit-ups<br>1min flutter kicks<br>2min rest \| 5 sets | **30**<br>10 minutes<br>side-to-side<br>leg raises<br>non-stop |

## 92 Touch Your Toes

Can't touch your toes? You are not alone. Good news, though, with a little bit of work it can be fixed! Warm up before doing the toe reach by doing leg swings and quad stretches. During this challenge you will first build up to a longer warm-up and then to a longer reach. The times for the warm-up are given in total so 30 seconds means 15 seconds per side. When performing the leg swings go for as wide swing as possible. You are warming up your hamstrings for the reach. When doing quad stretches bring your heels to your butt. And remember - you can do this! You should be able to see progress in the first 10 days.

# Touch Your Toes

## IN 30 DAYS CHALLENGE

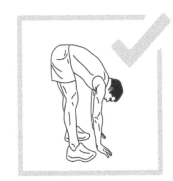

© darebee.com

| 1 | 2 | 3 | 4 | 5 |
|---|---|---|---|---|
| **30sec** leg swings<br>**30sec** quad stretch<br>**10sec** toe reach | **30sec** leg swings<br>**30sec** quad stretch<br>**10sec** toe reach | **30sec** leg swings<br>**30sec** quad stretch<br>**10sec** toe reach | **40sec** leg swings<br>**40sec** quad stretch<br>**15sec** toe reach | **40sec** leg swings<br>**40sec** quad stretch<br>**15sec** toe reach |

| 6 | 7 | 8 | 9 | 10 |
|---|---|---|---|---|
| **40sec** leg swings<br>**40sec** quad stretch<br>**15sec** toe reach | **60sec** leg swings<br>**60sec** quad stretch<br>**20sec** toe reach | **60sec** leg swings<br>**60sec** quad stretch<br>**20sec** toe reach | **60sec** leg swings<br>**60sec** quad stretch<br>**20sec** toe reach | **60sec** leg swings<br>**60sec** quad stretch<br>**25sec** toe reach |

| 11 | 12 | 13 | 14 | 15 |
|---|---|---|---|---|
| **60sec** leg swings<br>**60sec** quad stretch<br>**25sec** toe reach | **60sec** leg swings<br>**60sec** quad stretch<br>**25sec** toe reach | **60sec** leg swings<br>**60sec** quad stretch<br>**30sec** toe reach | **60sec** leg swings<br>**60sec** quad stretch<br>**30sec** toe reach | **60sec** leg swings<br>**60sec** quad stretch<br>**30sec** toe reach |

| 16 | 17 | 18 | 19 | 20 |
|---|---|---|---|---|
| **60sec** leg swings<br>**60sec** quad stretch<br>**35sec** toe reach | **60sec** leg swings<br>**60sec** quad stretch<br>**35sec** toe reach | **60sec** leg swings<br>**60sec** quad stretch<br>**35sec** toe reach | **60sec** leg swings<br>**60sec** quad stretch<br>**40sec** toe reach | **60sec** leg swings<br>**60sec** quad stretch<br>**40sec** toe reach |

| 21 | 22 | 23 | 24 | 25 |
|---|---|---|---|---|
| **60sec** leg swings<br>**60sec** quad stretch<br>**40sec** toe reach | **60sec** leg swings<br>**60sec** quad stretch<br>**45sec** toe reach | **60sec** leg swings<br>**60sec** quad stretch<br>**45sec** toe reach | **60sec** leg swings<br>**60sec** quad stretch<br>**45sec** toe reach | **60sec** leg swings<br>**60sec** quad stretch<br>**50sec** toe reach |

| 26 | 27 | 28 | 29 | 30 |
|---|---|---|---|---|
| **60sec** leg swings<br>**60sec** quad stretch<br>**50sec** toe reach | **60sec** leg swings<br>**60sec** quad stretch<br>**50sec** toe reach | **60sec** leg swings<br>**60sec** quad stretch<br>**60sec** toe reach | **60sec** leg swings<br>**60sec** quad stretch<br>**60sec** toe reach | **60sec** leg swings<br>**60sec** quad stretch<br>**60sec** toe reach |

## 93    Tricep Dips

Sculpt your upper body with the Tricep Dips Challenge! Targeted muscles: triceps and shoulders.

Instructions: Use a sofa, a chair or any type of knee-height ledge to perform tricep dips. Go as low as you can. To increase the difficulty, place a weight on your lap. Alternatively, you can do tricep dips without a ledge using a basic household floor.

# TRICEP DIPS

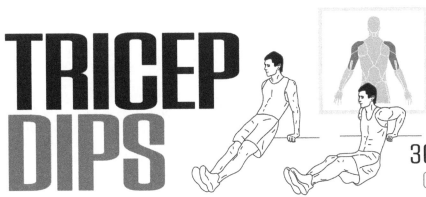

### 30-day challenge
© darebee.com

| | | | | |
|---|---|---|---|---|
| **1**<br>**6 tricep dips**<br>3 sets<br>30 seconds rest | **2**<br>**20 seconds**<br>tricep dip hold | **3**<br>**6 tricep dips**<br>4 sets<br>30 seconds rest | **4**<br>**20 seconds**<br>tricep dip hold | **5**<br>**8 tricep dips**<br>3 sets<br>30 seconds rest |
| **6**<br>**30 seconds**<br>tricep dip hold | **7**<br>**8 tricep dips**<br>4 sets<br>30 seconds rest | **8**<br>**30 seconds**<br>tricep dip hold | **9**<br>**10 tricep dips**<br>3 sets<br>30 seconds rest | **10**<br>**40 seconds**<br>tricep dip hold |
| **11**<br>**10 tricep dips**<br>4 sets<br>30 seconds rest | **12**<br>**40 seconds**<br>tricep dip hold | **13**<br>**12 tricep dips**<br>3 sets<br>30 seconds rest | **14**<br>**50 seconds**<br>tricep dip hold | **15**<br>**12 tricep dips**<br>4 sets<br>30 seconds rest |
| **16**<br>**50 seconds**<br>tricep dip hold | **17**<br>**14 tricep dips**<br>3 sets<br>30 seconds rest | **18**<br>**60 seconds**<br>tricep dip hold | **19**<br>**14 tricep dips**<br>4 sets<br>30 seconds rest | **20**<br>**60 seconds**<br>tricep dip hold |
| **21**<br>**16 tricep dips**<br>3 sets<br>30 seconds rest | **22**<br>**1min 10sec**<br>tricep dip hold | **23**<br>**16 tricep dips**<br>4 sets<br>30 seconds rest | **24**<br>**1min 10sec**<br>tricep dip hold | **25**<br>**18 tricep dips**<br>3 sets<br>30 seconds rest |
| **26**<br>**1min 20sec**<br>tricep dip hold | **27**<br>**18 tricep dips**<br>4 sets<br>30 seconds rest | **28**<br>**1min 20sec**<br>tricep dip hold | **29**<br>**20 tricep dips**<br>3 sets<br>30 seconds rest | **30**<br>**1min 30sec**<br>tricep dip hold |

# 94  Upper Body

Increase your upper body strength and, by extension, your overall athleticism with a challenge that incrementally helps you get stronger. The exercises, each day, build a cumulative load that triggers the body's adaptive response and helps you acquire stronger muscles.

You will feel different, walk differently and even tire less, as a result. Plus, the sheer dedication of training every day helps you build positive habits that help you in your life as well as your fitness.

# upper body

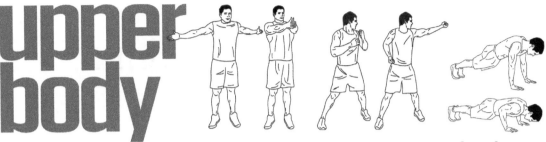

## 30-DAY CHALLENGE

© darebee.com

| 1 | 2 | 3 | 4 | 5 |
|---|---|---|---|---|
| 12 backfists<br>6 push-ups<br>3 sets \| 2 min rest | **40**<br>chest expansions<br>in total for the day | 12 backfists<br>6 push-ups<br>4 sets \| 2 min rest | **44**<br>chest expansions<br>in total for the day | 12 backfists<br>6 push-ups<br>5 sets \| 2 min rest |

| 6 | 7 | 8 | 9 | 10 |
|---|---|---|---|---|
| **48**<br>chest expansions<br>in total for the day | 16 backfists<br>8 push-ups<br>3 sets \| 2 min rest | **50**<br>chest expansions<br>in total for the day | 16 backfists<br>8 push-ups<br>4 sets \| 2 min rest | **52**<br>chest expansions<br>in total for the day |

| 11 | 12 | 13 | 14 | 15 |
|---|---|---|---|---|
| 16 backfists<br>8 push-ups<br>5 sets \| 2 min rest | **54**<br>chest expansions<br>in total for the day | 20 backfists<br>10 push-ups<br>3 sets \| 2 min rest | **56**<br>chest expansions<br>in total for the day | 20 backfists<br>10 push-ups<br>4 sets \| 2 min rest |

| 16 | 17 | 18 | 19 | 20 |
|---|---|---|---|---|
| **60**<br>chest expansions<br>in total for the day | 20 backfists<br>10 push-ups<br>5 sets \| 2 min rest | **64**<br>chest expansions<br>in total for the day | 24 backfists<br>12 push-ups<br>3 sets \| 2 min rest | **68**<br>chest expansions<br>in total for the day |

| 21 | 22 | 23 | 24 | 25 |
|---|---|---|---|---|
| 24 backfists<br>12 push-ups<br>4 sets \| 2 min rest | **72**<br>chest expansions<br>in total for the day | 24 backfists<br>12 push-ups<br>5 sets \| 2 min rest | **76**<br>chest expansions<br>in total for the day | 28 backfists<br>14 push-ups<br>3 sets \| 2 min rest |

| 26 | 27 | 28 | 29 | 30 |
|---|---|---|---|---|
| **80**<br>chest expansions<br>in total for the day | 28 backfists<br>14 push-ups<br>4 sets \| 2 min rest | **84**<br>chest expansions<br>in total for the day | 28 backfists<br>14 push-ups<br>5 sets \| 2 min rest | **88**<br>chest expansions<br>in total for the day |

## 95 Upper Body Light

Developing great upper body strength is a function of consistency, incremental load, variety and focus. The Upper Body Light Challenge provides an easy means to maintain some of the pressure required for muscular and neural adaptations to take place. It is an awesome addition to everything else you do on the days you exercise and a brilliant way to keep things revving on the days when you're too busy to get in a harder workout.

Instructions: Keep your arms up during a set.

# upper body LIGHT

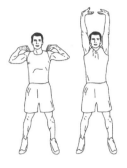
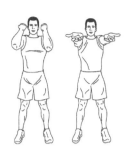
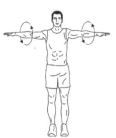

## 30-DAY CHALLENGE

© darebee.com

| | | | | |
|---|---|---|---|---|
| **1**<br>40 shoulder taps<br>40 bicep extensions<br>3 sets \| 30sec rest | **2**<br>**60**<br>raised arm circles<br>in one go | **3**<br>40 shoulder taps<br>40 bicep extensions<br>3 sets \| 30sec rest | **4**<br>**80**<br>raised arm circles<br>in one go | **5**<br>40 shoulder taps<br>40 bicep extensions<br>3 sets \| 30sec rest |
| **6**<br>**100**<br>raised arm circles<br>in one go | **7**<br>50 shoulder taps<br>50 bicep extensions<br>3 sets \| 30sec rest | **8**<br>**120**<br>raised arm circles<br>in one go | **9**<br>50 shoulder taps<br>50 bicep extensions<br>3 sets \| 30sec rest | **10**<br>**140**<br>raised arm circles<br>in one go |
| **11**<br>50 shoulder taps<br>50 bicep extensions<br>3 sets \| 30sec rest | **12**<br>**160**<br>raised arm circles<br>in one go | **13**<br>60 shoulder taps<br>60 bicep extensions<br>3 sets \| 30sec rest | **14**<br>**180**<br>raised arm circles<br>in one go | **15**<br>60 shoulder taps<br>60 bicep extensions<br>3 sets \| 30sec rest |
| **16**<br>**200**<br>raised arm circles<br>in one go | **17**<br>60 shoulder taps<br>60 bicep extensions<br>3 sets \| 30sec rest | **18**<br>**220**<br>raised arm circles<br>in one go | **19**<br>70 shoulder taps<br>70 bicep extensions<br>3 sets \| 30sec rest | **20**<br>**240**<br>raised arm circles<br>in one go |
| **21**<br>70 shoulder taps<br>70 bicep extensions<br>3 sets \| 30sec rest | **22**<br>**260**<br>raised arm circles<br>in one go | **23**<br>70 shoulder taps<br>70 bicep extensions<br>3 sets \| 30sec rest | **24**<br>**280**<br>raised arm circles<br>in one go | **25**<br>80 shoulder taps<br>80 bicep extensions<br>3 sets \| 30sec rest |
| **26**<br>**300**<br>raised arm circles<br>in one go | **27**<br>80 shoulder taps<br>80 bicep extensions<br>3 sets \| 30sec rest | **28**<br>**320**<br>raised arm circles<br>in one go | **29**<br>80 shoulder taps<br>80 bicep extensions<br>3 sets \| 30sec rest | **30**<br>**340**<br>raised arm circles<br>in one go |

## 96 | Upper Body Plus

Training the upper body requires dedication, patience and perseverance or, the more usually cited three Ps of perspiration, patience and perseverance. The good news here is that there is very little perspiration involved in this challenge.

Each set of exercises, each day, is short enough to just get you feeling a little warm. Yet, collectively they deliver a change to your upper body strength that will be noticeable by the end of the month.

# upper body+

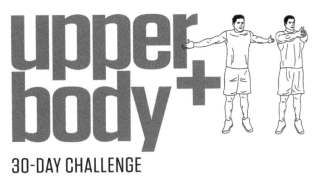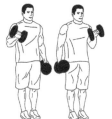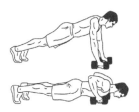

## 30-DAY CHALLENGE

© darebee.com

| | | | | |
|---|---|---|---|---|
| **1**<br>6 bicep curls<br>6 push-ups<br>3 sets \| 2 min rest | **2**<br>40<br>chest expansions<br>in total for the day | **3**<br>6 bicep curls<br>6 push-ups<br>4 sets \| 2 min rest | **4**<br>44<br>chest expansions<br>in total for the day | **5**<br>6 bicep curls<br>6 push-ups<br>5 sets \| 2 min rest |
| **6**<br>48<br>chest expansions<br>in total for the day | **7**<br>8 bicep curls<br>8 push-ups<br>3 sets \| 2 min rest | **8**<br>50<br>chest expansions<br>in total for the day | **9**<br>8 bicep curls<br>8 push-ups<br>4 sets \| 2 min rest | **10**<br>52<br>chest expansions<br>in total for the day |
| **11**<br>8 bicep curls<br>8 push-ups<br>5 sets \| 2 min rest | **12**<br>54<br>chest expansions<br>in total for the day | **13**<br>10 bicep curls<br>10 push-ups<br>3 sets \| 2 min rest | **14**<br>56<br>chest expansions<br>in total for the day | **15**<br>10 bicep curls<br>10 push-ups<br>4 sets \| 2 min rest |
| **16**<br>60<br>chest expansions<br>in total for the day | **17**<br>10 bicep curls<br>10 push-ups<br>5 sets \| 2 min rest | **18**<br>64<br>chest expansions<br>in total for the day | **19**<br>12 bicep curls<br>12 push-ups<br>3 sets \| 2 min rest | **20**<br>68<br>chest expansions<br>in total for the day |
| **21**<br>12 bicep curls<br>12 push-ups<br>4 sets \| 2 min rest | **22**<br>72<br>chest expansions<br>in total for the day | **23**<br>12 bicep curls<br>12 push-ups<br>5 sets \| 2 min rest | **24**<br>76<br>chest expansions<br>in total for the day | **25**<br>14 bicep curls<br>14 push-ups<br>3 sets \| 2 min rest |
| **26**<br>80<br>chest expansions<br>in total for the day | **27**<br>14 bicep curls<br>14 push-ups<br>4 sets \| 2 min rest | **28**<br>84<br>chest expansions<br>in total for the day | **29**<br>14 bicep curls<br>14 push-ups<br>5 sets \| 2 min rest | **30**<br>88<br>chest expansions<br>in total for the day |

## 97   Walkabout

Walking keeps your body active, your blood stream oxygenated and your brain alert. Scientific studies have shown that the seemingly simple impact of your foot on the ground, as you walk, is sufficient to activate higher function centers in the brain and make thinking clearer. This, in turn, has been shown to positively impact IQ points.

Take up a 30-day walkabout challenge and make your every step count. Use a pedometer or a free mobile app to track your progress throughout the day.

# 30 DAY
# WALKABOUT

CHALLENGE    split total steps into manageable sets

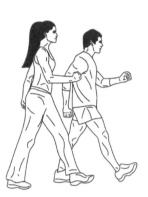

© darebee.com

| | | | | |
|---|---|---|---|---|
| **1**<br>5,000<br>steps | **2**<br>5,500<br>steps | **3**<br>6,000<br>steps | **4**<br>5,000<br>steps | **5**<br>6,500<br>steps |
| **6**<br>7,000<br>steps | **7**<br>7,500<br>steps | **8**<br>5,000<br>steps | **9**<br>8,000<br>steps | **10**<br>8,500<br>steps |
| **11**<br>9,000<br>steps | **12**<br>5,000<br>steps | **13**<br>9,500<br>steps | **14**<br>10,000<br>steps | **15**<br>10,500<br>steps |
| **16**<br>5,000<br>steps | **17**<br>11,000<br>steps | **18**<br>11,500<br>steps | **19**<br>12,000<br>steps | **20**<br>5,000<br>steps |
| **21**<br>12,500<br>steps | **22**<br>13,000<br>steps | **23**<br>13,500<br>steps | **24**<br>5,000<br>steps | **25**<br>14,000<br>steps |
| **26**<br>14,500<br>steps | **27**<br>15,000<br>steps | **28**<br>5,000<br>steps | **29**<br>15,500<br>steps | **30**<br>16,000<br>steps |

## 98 Wall Push-Ups

Push-ups have the potential to change your entire body. They affect core, glutes, quads, abs, chest, shoulders, back and triceps. We all have to start from somewhere which is why the Wall Push-Up Challenge becomes the proofing ground you need to prepare you for your fitness journey. Through 30 days you will feel the transformation.

Instructions: For the wall push-up hold to failure lower yourself into a wall push-up position and hold it for as long as you can, even if it's just 5 seconds. Repeat 3 times in total with a 30 second break in between.

# wall push-ups

## 30-DAY CHALLENGE

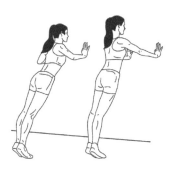

© darebee.com

| | | | | |
|---|---|---|---|---|
| **1**<br>**12 wall push-ups**<br>5 sets<br>30 seconds rest | **2**<br>**wall push-up hold**<br>3 sets **to failure**<br>30 seconds rest | **3**<br>**12 wall push-ups**<br>5 sets<br>30 seconds rest | **4**<br>**wall push-up hold**<br>3 sets **to failure**<br>30 seconds rest | **5**<br>**12 wall push-ups**<br>5 sets<br>30 seconds rest |
| **6**<br>**wall push-up hold**<br>3 sets **to failure**<br>30 seconds rest | **7**<br>**14 wall push-ups**<br>5 sets<br>30 seconds rest | **8**<br>**wall push-up hold**<br>3 sets **to failure**<br>30 seconds rest | **9**<br>**14 wall push-ups**<br>5 sets<br>30 seconds rest | **10**<br>**wall push-up hold**<br>3 sets **to failure**<br>30 seconds rest |
| **11**<br>**14 wall push-ups**<br>5 sets<br>30 seconds rest | **12**<br>**wall push-up hold**<br>3 sets **to failure**<br>30 seconds rest | **13**<br>**16 wall push-ups**<br>5 sets<br>30 seconds rest | **14**<br>**wall push-up hold**<br>3 sets **to failure**<br>30 seconds rest | **15**<br>**16 wall push-ups**<br>5 sets<br>30 seconds rest |
| **16**<br>**wall push-up hold**<br>3 sets **to failure**<br>30 seconds rest | **17**<br>**16 wall push-ups**<br>5 sets<br>30 seconds rest | **18**<br>**wall push-up hold**<br>3 sets **to failure**<br>30 seconds rest | **19**<br>**18 wall push-ups**<br>5 sets<br>30 seconds rest | **20**<br>**wall push-up hold**<br>3 sets **to failure**<br>30 seconds rest |
| **21**<br>**18 wall push-ups**<br>5 sets<br>30 seconds rest | **22**<br>**wall push-up hold**<br>3 sets **to failure**<br>30 seconds rest | **23**<br>**18 wall push-ups**<br>5 sets<br>30 seconds rest | **24**<br>**wall push-up hold**<br>3 sets **to failure**<br>30 seconds rest | **25**<br>**20 wall push-ups**<br>5 sets<br>30 seconds rest |
| **26**<br>**wall push-up hold**<br>3 sets **to failure**<br>30 seconds rest | **27**<br>**20 wall push-ups**<br>5 sets<br>30 seconds rest | **28**<br>**wall push-up hold**<br>3 sets **to failure**<br>30 seconds rest | **29**<br>**20 wall push-ups**<br>5 sets<br>30 seconds rest | **30**<br>**wall push-up hold**<br>3 sets **to failure**<br>30 seconds rest |

## 99    Wall-Sit

Wall Sit is an exercise that pits the power of your quads and the ability of your brain to focus and not give in to fatigue against the gravity of the planet, trying to drag you down.

To succeed you have to fight gravity on a daily basis for incrementally increasing periods of time. The reward for your efforts are noticeably stronger legs and a mind that can focus sufficiently to overcome the limitations of the body.

# WALL-SIT

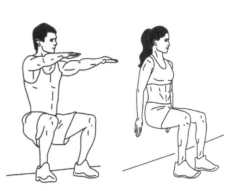

## 30-DAY CHALLENGE © darebee.com

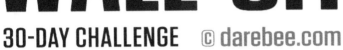

| | | | | |
|---|---|---|---|---|
| **1**<br>**20 seconds**<br>wall-sit | **2**<br>**30 seconds**<br>wall-sit | **3**<br>**40 seconds**<br>wall-sit | **4**<br>**20 seconds**<br>wall-sit | **5**<br>**50 seconds**<br>wall-sit |
| **6**<br>**60 seconds**<br>wall-sit | **7**<br>**1min 10sec**<br>wall-sit | **8**<br>**20 seconds**<br>wall-sit | **9**<br>**1min 20sec**<br>wall-sit | **10**<br>**1min 30sec**<br>wall-sit |
| **11**<br>**1min 40sec**<br>wall-sit | **12**<br>**20 seconds**<br>wall-sit | **13**<br>**1min 50sec**<br>wall-sit | **14**<br>**2 minutes**<br>wall-sit | **15**<br>**2min 10sec**<br>wall-sit |
| **16**<br>**20 seconds**<br>wall-sit | **17**<br>**2min 20sec**<br>wall-sit | **18**<br>**2min 30sec**<br>wall-sit | **19**<br>**2min 40sec**<br>wall-sit | **20**<br>**20 seconds**<br>wall-sit |
| **21**<br>**2min 50sec**<br>wall-sit | **22**<br>**3 minutes**<br>wall-sit | **23**<br>**3min 10sec**<br>wall-sit | **24**<br>**20 seconds**<br>wall-sit | **25**<br>**3min 20sec**<br>wall-sit |
| **26**<br>**3min 30sec**<br>wall-sit | **27**<br>**3min 40sec**<br>wall-sit | **28**<br>**20 seconds**<br>wall-sit | **29**<br>**3min 50sec**<br>wall-sit | **30**<br>**4 minutes**<br>wall-sit |

## 100 Yoga Abs

As the difficulty of the challenge increases throughout the 30 days you are guaranteed to feel every second of it. During the final five seconds of each set is when you will be gaining the most. Try to keep it up! It'll be worth it.

Instructions: Add this challenge to your everyday training at the end of your session. It'll make an ideal finisher. After the boat pose hold, slowly transition to knee hug and hold it for the same amount of time. Transition like this 3 times in total (3 sets) to complete the challenge for the day. Don't forget to tighten your core, if you can. If you can't, it's not quite there yet but that's why you are working on it! With consistency and determination you will feel and see your abs in no time. Use the custom timer above to set the time.

Tip: To make the challenge harder change the boat hold to hollow hold. It'll increase the difficulty and subsequently improve the end result.

# yoga abs

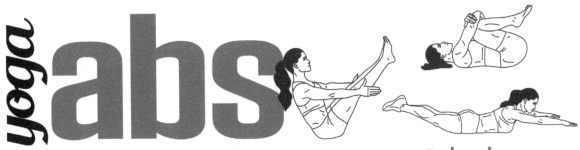

## 30-DAY CHALLENGE

© darebee.com

| | | | | |
|---|---|---|---|---|
| **1**<br>**20sec** boat pose<br>**20sec** knee hug<br>3 sets | **2**<br>**20sec** superman<br>**20sec** rest<br>3 sets | **3**<br>**20sec** boat pose<br>**20sec** knee hug<br>3 sets | **4**<br>**20sec** superman<br>**20sec** rest<br>3 sets | **5**<br>**25sec** boat pose<br>**25sec** knee hug<br>3 sets |
| **6**<br>**25sec** superman<br>**25sec** rest<br>3 sets | **7**<br>**25sec** boat pose<br>**25sec** knee hug<br>3 sets | **8**<br>**25sec** superman<br>**25sec** rest<br>3 sets | **9**<br>**30sec** boat pose<br>**30sec** knee hug<br>3 sets | **10**<br>**30sec** superman<br>**30sec** rest<br>3 sets |
| **11**<br>**30sec** boat pose<br>**30sec** knee hug<br>3 sets | **12**<br>**30sec** superman<br>**30sec** rest<br>3 sets | **13**<br>**35sec** boat pose<br>**35sec** knee hug<br>3 sets | **14**<br>**35sec** superman<br>**35sec** rest<br>3 sets | **15**<br>**35sec** boat pose<br>**35sec** knee hug<br>3 sets |
| **16**<br>**35sec** superman<br>**35sec** rest<br>3 sets | **17**<br>**40sec** boat pose<br>**40sec** knee hug<br>3 sets | **18**<br>**40sec** superman<br>**40sec** rest<br>3 sets | **19**<br>**40sec** boat pose<br>**40sec** knee hug<br>3 sets | **20**<br>**40sec** superman<br>**40sec** rest<br>3 sets |
| **21**<br>**45sec** boat pose<br>**45sec** knee hug<br>3 sets | **22**<br>**45sec** superman<br>**45sec** rest<br>3 sets | **23**<br>**45sec** boat pose<br>**45sec** knee hug<br>3 sets | **24**<br>**45sec** superman<br>**45sec** rest<br>3 sets | **25**<br>**50sec** boat pose<br>**50sec** knee hug<br>3 sets |
| **26**<br>**50sec** superman<br>**50sec** rest<br>3 sets | **27**<br>**50sec** boat pose<br>**50sec** knee hug<br>3 sets | **28**<br>**50sec** superman<br>**50sec** rest<br>3 sets | **29**<br>**60sec** boat pose<br>**60sec** knee hug<br>3 sets | **30**<br>**60sec** superman<br>**60sec** rest<br>3 sets |

CPSIA information can be obtained
at www.ICGtesting.com
Printed in the USA
BVHW010144160222
629082BV00006B/405